ANCIENT AND MODERN SECRETS OF

HEALTH AND LONG LIFE

ALTERNATIVE MEDICINE, ALTERNATIVE

THERAPIES AND ALTERNATIVE HEALTH

BY DR. LAURA ZEAMAN

ACKNOWLEDGEMENTS

This book is dedicated to my husband and all the patients who voluntarily partook in my experiments during the creation of this book. A special thanks to you all.

TABLE OF CONTENT

5

1. INTRODUCTION

In our world today, anti-aging products (cosmetics and drugs) and procedures are a multi-billion-dollar business. Why? No one wants to look that faded, wrinkled or old. People will practically pay anything to look younger, preserve youthfulness and vitality. But slow as she moves, old Mother Time catches up with everyone sooner or later.

But, hey! Before you get all upset and miserable, read on a bit....

Does getting older mean you are less important in society? Does it mean you are less valuable, or even less beautiful? Not at all, the contrary is even the case. Ever heard of the term 'Graceful Aging"?

Aging can actually be delightful, it's certainly a dignified process if handled right. As you age, with the right knowledge and habits, you can slow things down a whole lot and actually enjoy the unique journey of longevity. More times than not, a person ends up more beautiful than he or she was when younger. Certainly, the person gets smarter and more valuable.

You see, when a young individual, male or female, is youthful, attractive and beautiful, it's really nice to behold, but definitely, no big deal as such things are quite commonplace. The real stunner is someone who is older but still beautiful and attractive with moist skin, firm flesh and an easy moving body. Now that's rare and quite phenomenal, as such, it has heads turning, attracting attention from every direction. On this note, let's take a look at the things you can do to bring about a more youthful and attractive look, vibrant complexion, vitality and superb general health in your body.

Yes, people want to live forever and remain young all the way. But one important thing they fail to understand about this is that all what they seek is merely a side effect of good health, which is the result of careful living and eating habits.

You are what you eat and how you live. Your body, (particularly your skin) reflects exactly what's going on inside your body and all around you. Have you got chronic skin problems, like wrinkles? You are a victim of environmental pollution, excessive exposure to sunlight or you just do not eat the proper foods. Do you have bad sight? You are not eating vitamin A rich foods. If it is heart disease, excessive weight gain or general body weakness, then the problem is more a lack of regular exercise than anything else, poor eating habits merely complicates matter a lot.

The situation now begs the question, what sort of foods do you eat to supply your body with needed nourishment? What habits do you have that only accelerates the aging process in your body? What do you do or think about for most of the day? What are your stress levels most of the time? What activities do you engage in to keep your body fit, strong and agile?

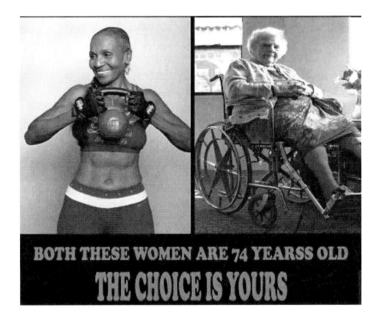

BOTH THESE WOMEN ARE 74 YEARSS OLD
THE CHOICE IS YOURS

Indeed, the choice is really yours to make – how you have life and live it.

Take a good look at your lifestyle right now by giving careful answers to the 5 simple questions. See if you're doing anything that's putting a strain on your body, thus aging it faster than it normally would.

Did you get all the wrong answers? Well, you don't need to go running off to a doctor or a drugstore just yet. Relax and read on. You are about to learn some simple but unique things you can start doing today and reap the benefits massively tomorrow, health wise. These things will help you defy even sequential (normal) aging in terms of how wonderful you look.

2. AGING, ANTI-AGING, HEALTH, LIFESPAN, AND LONGEVITY

These are all major terminologies (or processes) under the subject of sequential aging. In a way, they are all interconnected and too repeatedly mentioned where the subject of aging is concerned so it is very necessary we define and clarify each term at this time before proceeding further.

Aging

Aging, also spelled ageing, with respect to humans, is the process of becoming older.

The human body actually ages in a micro way every second, right from birth, and so aging can best be defined as a representation of the accumulation of changes in a human being over time. These changes take place on different levels – physical, psychological, and social levels. Up to a point, these changes are mostly positive and welcome, but beyond that, they are generally negative, very much unwelcome, and too often lead to death.

13

Anti-Aging

Anti-aging, is the careful process of fighting, slowing down or halting aging to a major degree. This complex process is executed at cellular levels and it leaves the body looking much younger and healthier – feeling it too.

The anti-aging process is made possible by the regular consumption of special foods and supplements, particularly designed by nature for the purpose. A new lifestyle and certain habits also play major roles in facilitating the anti-aging process,

The anti-aging process is basically a war to be fought every day, and the enemy is aging, which destroys your body from the inside out, using the powerful weapons of disease, harmful chemicals, free radicals, and toxins, which all get in your body mostly through the polluted environment and bad foods.

Thanks to nature, the war of anti-aging is not a very difficult one. It has been called interesting, even delicious (due to the associating foods), but one thing is for certain, the rewards are worth any trouble several times over.

Lifespan

Lifespan, with respect to humans, is defined as the predictable length of a person's life or the length of time a person can be expected to remain alive.

An increase in the lifespan of someone or a collective group of people such as a tribe simply means an increase in the days that person or group of people are expected to live or tend to live. Of note here is that while an individual's lifespan may increase (i.e. from 70 to 100 years), there are no guarantees that the individual must live up to the predicted number of years (i.e. 100 years) because there is always the issue of premature death – accidental death, death by sickness or disease, or even murder. Without the issue of premature death cutting short the individual's natural life, the person will live to the full duration of his or her lifespan, probably more.

Longevity

Longevity (long life) or the duration of life, refers to the length of an individual's life. The two, longevity and lifespan, are somewhat similar but not quite. Longevity is not to be mistaken for lifespan.

Longevity is the length of time a person has actually lived or is guaranteed to live while lifespan is the length of time a person is expected to live – and this is why you find the term '**longevity**' or '**long life**' used by most companies in the marketing of their products. They refer to a guarantee of lengthy durability.

A person (or group of people i.e. a family or tribe) who tend to live to, let's say, 120 years are said to have unusual longevity (or unusual long life). However, when that person was much younger, based on certain factors, the person may be said to have a long lifespan (expected to live a long time or last a long time) – or shorter lifespan in the case of the discovery of a life-threatening chronic disease like cancer.

Longevity is a proven or guaranteed period of durability but lifespan is merely a prediction of durability.

Health

There are various degrees of good health but perfect health is what you want because it alone guarantees a disease-free life and longevity. Only with the right foods and lifestyle can you attain good health, but if gone about very correctly and dedicatedly, then **perfect health** is the reward.

Health is the connection between all four subjects above – aging, anti-aging, lifespan, and longevity. While **Aging** fosters bad health in the body, the counter process of **anti-aging** fosters good health. Longevity (long life), or a major increase in lifespan, is as a direct result of **perfect health**, not just good health, – it is a victorious anti-aging war!

Allowing aging creep up on you the wrong way – without proper control – will wreak havoc in your body and destroy what little good health you have. One way or another, with time, it will lead to death.

Ever heard of the term '**accelerated aging**'? Ever seen a person of 40 who looks 60 or a person of 60 who looks 100? Ever seen a middle-aged person suffering from more health complications than you can count on the fingers of both hands, most of it incurable illnesses and diseases? In today's world, full of pollution and bad foods as it is, accelerated aging, which leads invariably to horrible health complications, is the case with our bodies. We do not age normally anymore but at a faster rate and the effects are hugely and completely negative, which translates to bad health and shorter lifespans. This is the major reason people lived longer lives in the past – when foods and the environment were clean – than they do today. Indeed, longevity is more a thing of the past now.

Anti-aging procedures are the only way to achieve perfect health, and consequently, long life. Fighting and controlling the aging process is what it takes and this is something you must do every day, post prime. If gotten right, longer life, youthfulness, and superb health are the rewards.

OTHER IMPORTANT TERMS RELATING TO AGING

Some other important terms or names relating to anti-aging and frequently mentioned in this book are explained below.

Antioxidants

This term refers to a unique group of powerful substances with the ability to inhibit or halt the negative and highly destructive effects of the body's oxidation processes, which does massive damages to cells and tissues over time.

All that oxygen you breathe in doesn't just do your body good, it does a whole lot of harm too, and this shows with time. Oxidation is the number one cause of accelerated aging in human beings, and as such, anti-antioxidants are so important to the anti-aging war.

Antioxidants can only be gotten from certain foods and supplements, and they differ depending on the source.

Free Radicals

Free radicals are very harmful compounds with extremely reactive groups of molecules or atoms that wreak havoc on the cells and tissues of the body.

Free radicals get in the body from the polluted environment and bad foods.

Toxins

Toxins are poisonous substances within the body. They are subdivided into two categories.

1. Poison formed by living organisms in the body.

2. Harmful substances that find their way into the body from the polluted environment.

Both kinds of toxins, if not flushed out of the body, tend to accumulate in the body over time.

Most of these poisons and harmful substances are usually removed by natural body detox processes but there are those that require more powerful methods to dislodge. The most common method to trigger the body's natural detox process is by drinking a lot of water. This helps the body flush out most of these toxins through the urine and sweat.

For more powerful detox procedures, certain health friendly compounds such as antioxidants are required. These and more are talked about in this book.

3. WHY THE HUGE CONCERN OVER AGING.

The saying goes "growing older is not for the timid". The wrinkles begin to form on the skin, hair colors lighten up on the way to gray, and the age starts to show around the eyes and mouths. Reaction time and agility slow down, and the body begins to weaken, memory begins to fade and disorientation sets in, age spots show up on the face and hands, and the anxiety mounts within us as time marches on.

While brain capacity, knowledge of world events and wisdom may expand, the many other effects of aging doesn't make it welcome. Aging is considered by many experts as the number one risk factor for most diseases and illnesses. Going by the current world statistics of numerous world health monitoring organizations, no less than 180,000 people die each day around the world, and well over two-thirds of these deaths are directly linked to age-related causes.

The worry about countering aging is not just to look good or younger but to live easier and happier, for as long as possible – a disease-free life.

4. THE PRIME IS THE LIMIT

The human 'prime' is the age at which the physical performance of the body peaks (reaches the highest level attainable).

From childhood to about thirty, the effects of aging are mostly positive. A human being reaches the prime of life at about thirty, most times two years before. After thirty, the negative side of aging sets in and life is no longer the same. From this period onwards, general body functions and organ performance begins to slow or fail.

Interestingly, it is very possible to retain most of the body's physical vitality and agility till well into the 30s and so a lot of people tend to remain in their sexual prime till 40, and sometimes, a few years beyond. But after that, overall body performance begins to deteriorate in earnest. Health problems such as skin wrinkles, eye problems, physical fitness issues, sexual dysfunction, become major problems once a person begins to age, post-prime. If not brought swiftly under control, these problems could escalate, leading to accelerated aging.

In the world of competitive sports and athletics where full fitness is a necessary requirement, it is a well-recognized fact that an athlete's performances peaks between the ages of 27 – 30 years, and then, begins to drop very visibly until eventual retirement soon after.

It is now a medically proven and universally accepted fact that the human body reaches its highest levels of overall performance at 28 years of age. From that point onwards, overall body performance begins to drop markedly.

Football, or soccer as the ball game is known in the United States and Canada, is one of the most popular sports in the world. It is a very entertaining, money rich sport, which requires players be at full fitness levels, and so professional football clubs, particularly the multimillion dollar clubs in Europe, never sign deals with footballers over 28 years of age unless they are exceptionally talented, uniquely fit and dedicated to training. Even then, the most such a footballer could ever hope for is a short 3-year deal, and after that, however, well he has performed. a one-year deal is all that is offered. Why? This is because these profit-minded clubs, and everyone else for that matter, are all too aware that, however gifted, a player's performance begins to deteriorate at after 28 years of age. At 31, the player's best days are gone and he merely gets worse daily, struggling for fitness all the way till 35, when he is finally forced to retire due to the overwhelming effects the aging process that slows down agility and response time.

The age of 28 is the prime of human beings. Once past that age, a human being's body is never physically the same again because the negative side of aging has finally set in.

From 28 and beyond, is the period to start giving anti-aging strategies serious thought. If a person chooses to start doing this much earlier, the better. Indulging regularly in simple anti-aging procedures, pre-prime, will extend the period of a person's prime well into the 30s.

5. CAUSES OF NORMAL AGING & ACCELERATED AGING

Normal Aging

The causes of normal aging in humans are still unclear to scientists. One theory, called the damage concept, has it that the accumulation of damage (e.g. DNA oxidation) may cause the human biological systems to fail. Another theory has it that the programmed aging concept, wherein internal processes (e.g. DNA telomere shortening) may cause aging.

Of note here is that programmed aging should not be confused with the integral process of programmed cell death (apoptosis), nor should the normal aging process be confused with accelerated aging.

Accelerated Aging

Accelerated aging is brought on by different factors including illnesses, diseases and pollution of the environment (the main way damaging free radicals get in the body), and the action of the sun's ultraviolet rays on the skin. Other factors that accelerate the aging process include lack of proper exercise, stress, and unhealthy eating and living habits.

As pointed out before, accelerated aging is the manner in which our body now ages and it's obviously due to so much environmental pollution, stress, and bad foods present around us today. Still, the entire aging process can be slowed and even halted in certain unique ways.

At 50, one could look the age, look 20 years younger or 20 years older. It all depends on how you age, or rather, how you control the process of aging in your body.

6. THE AGE-OLD ANTI-AGING WAR

How do I stop the process of aging in my body? How do I slow aging and look younger? These questions have been on the tongues and minds of millions and millions of people around the world for generations.

The unique discovery, in 1934, that the restriction of calorie in the body could extend lifespan by 50% in rats, a spice of mammals similar to humans in many ways, has motivated direct research into delaying and preventing aging in human beings.

Another angle of research pursued by scientists is that of simple and healthy living. People the world over have come to realize that mountains of expensive modern drugs and medication don't necessarily guarantee good health, long life and youthfulness, whereas, clean and simple living habits, paired up with careful eating habits does.

Proof Man Can Live To 900 years

According to the HOLY BIBLE of Christianity, there was a time when human beings lived up to and beyond 900 years of age. The first man created by God, Adam, lived to

150 years before he had his child with his wife, Eve. Adam is said to have lived up to 930 years, begetting sons and daughters all the way, before he died. Seth, Adam's third son, lived 105 years before he begot his first son, Enosh. Seth lived a total of 912 years, putting forth more sons and daughters before he died. And Enosh, on his part, lived to 905 years before he died….

And so, the genealogy of the descendants of the first man, Adam, went on in the opening chapters of the Bible book of Genesis, with a long record of people with incredible longevity. Such a thing as a person living over 150 years seems like a bad joke today, what with the average life expectancy in some countries coming in as low as 40 years, with people looking like ancient vegetable at 70. However, when one considers that at the dawn of creation, or evolution as scientists see it, human beings lived lives in the cleanest and healthiest of ways; everything they consumed was very clean, pure and rich – water, food (fruits and vegetable eaten mostly raw daily) – even the air was so clean and pure, and harmful things like pollution, bacteria, illnesses, and diseases did not even exist then! Add all these to the fact that life was a lot less stressful at the time and vigorous exercise routines on a daily basis was a given as everyone had to move around on foot and literality do his or her own work, and the whole angle of living extraordinary long lives at the dawn of creation begins to make some sense.

Introducing the Golden Secret of Anti-aging

In this book, we will take a good look at some of these clean and healthy ways of life that promote longevity; the unique foods and excise routines that can help fight, slow or even halt the aging process in human beings to a marked degree. We will also look at rare and odd solutions to stopping the unwelcome aging process, some dating back hundreds of years. Among these rare and odd solutions lies a little-known secret, so effective in fighting the aging process that it even halts it to a major extent. This secret which I will share in this book is known to some knowledgeable individuals as the **GOLDEN SECRET OF ANTI-AGING**.

Yes, there are quite a few great secrets when it comes to anti-aging strategies. With origins in different cultures and traditions spread over generations, most of these secrets will amaze you, but none of them, not even the best modern remedies available in the world today, comes even close to equaling this **GOLDEN SECRET** in effectiveness.

7. THE BEST ANTI-AGING STRATEGIES

You've heard it said a billion and one times before but I'll repeat anyway: You are exactly what you eat. Yes, by your diet alone you can delay or even shut down certain aging process in your body.

How wonderful it is to behold a lovely and attractive woman of 60 who looks 20 years younger, or a youthful! looking man of 70 who competes actively in a marathon race, most amazing of all is a very healthy man in his 60s with an active sex life! Don't be surprised, all these and more can be accomplished with the proper anti-aging strategy which merely entails eating the right diets and undergoing the right exercise routines for short periods daily. This strategy works best when started early enough in life, well before the aging process really sets in. Once the negative aspects of aging set in during middle-age, there is no going back no matter what you do. Prevention is the only opinion here as a cure for aging is not currently a possibility. Improving your diet today, while you still have much youthfulness in your body to preserve, is the number one step in the right direction: this will slow down the aging process, and thus preserve that youthfulness in you.

Let's face the harsh truth: while modern medical treatments (i.e. cosmetic surgery and the likes of it) may improve your appearance, it will not solve the problems that originally led to the skin wrinkles, sagging flesh, failing immune system and organs. We may be able to beautify ourselves with modern procedures but without supplying the body with the right minerals and nutrients, without the right living habits, all that beauty will waste away, and quickly too!

It's now time to adapt an anti-aging strategy in your life – one that will rejuvenate the body thoroughly from the inside out, guaranteeing vitality, superb health, and nourishment.

8. IMPORTANT TIPS FOR A NEW STRATEGY AND LIFESTYLE

What Are You Eating in your diet?

A good meal is certainly not enough, regularly eating a balanced diet: one full of nutrients and vitamins is what you need – what your body needs. Foods that protect the body against diseases and help it fight the aging process is what you should consume on a daily basis. Many minor health conditions are merely warning signs that you are doing something wrong or simply not doing the right thing. With regards to eating the right foods, look first to your skin, the largest organ in the body which performs so many vital tasks to keep you healthy. If by your eating habits your body is deficient in, say, vitamins and minerals, your system, triggered by brain commands, will take care of your more vital organs (liver and heart) first, and so your skin (nails and hair) will suffer. If you are deficient in just vitamin A, your skin will suffer first before you eye sight gets affected next. With a deficiency in the important omega-3 fats, your skin will lose its fresh, and moist look before the first signs of, say, heart problems set in.

Wait! Do not go running scared to see the doctor, you do not need him just yet. There are many verities of nutrient rich food you can add to your diet right now and see changes in your body within a few short hours. They are all delicious and easy to prepare too! These foods are dealt with in detail in the book.

How much sleep do you get?

A good night's rest or sleep is one of the best things you can do for yourself. It lowers brains stress levels and prevents accelerated aging too. This aspect of the anti-aging fight is one of the most overlooked health habits. Pick a dark cool room and go to sleep – try to get some good sleep for at least 8 hours each day.

How Sweet A Tooth Do You Have?

We are talking the amount of sugar and sugary stuff you consume each day. The average American consumes more than 100 pounds of sugar per year!!! That's quite a lot but very understandable because sugar is in almost everything Americans eat– from snickerdoodles to soda. If you live in the United States, sugar is something that's very difficult to avoid. Unfortunately, sugar is the number one substance that accelerates (fuels) the aging process in the human body.

Do you want a healthy and youthful body with nice skin? You should start avoiding sugar at all costs today.

That harmless looking white stuff you shovel into your foods actually comes as an unattractive brown natural substance and so bleach is used to whiten it up attractively. Is bleach something you want in your body or food? I think not. Sugar is very acidic once in the body and so doesn't do your health one bit of good. Sugar is completely devoid of nutrients and so is classified as an "empty calorie". Poor health is all you get from that fine white stuff called sugar and strangely enough, it can just be as addictive as hard drugs – you always end up wanting more and more of it.

To preserve your health, your precious skin and waistline, dump the sugar already. Are you already hooked onto sugar addiction? Asking you to dump sugar is like asking you to stop breathing, right? Well, never fear. All that's need is an adjustment and you'll be fine, much better even.

The trick here is to find a substitute as sweet as sugar but not sugar. Maple syrup or coconut nectar are very good options, but pure natural honey beats both. Honey is simply incredible because, though, unprocessed, is so sweet and it even contains vital minerals, nutrients, and enzymes. That honey is more satisfying and even sweeter than sugar is a fact many can testify to, so you don't need that much of it. Time to get rid of that sugar now and go shopping for a big bottle of pure natural honey.

What Is Your Skin Eating?

Yes, it's quite true that your skin eats. Since it absorbs whatever you rub on it or spray on it, your skin actually eats, absorbing it all into your body. In this regard, if you use skin care products that contain harmful chemicals, then those harmful chemicals are being absorbed directly into your body. On the average, a woman absorbs about five pounds of chemicals into her body from her makeup products alone each year. Why not use organic products which help with anti-aging? These products can even be mixed in with your regular cosmetics.

What organic products? There are quite a few – olive oil, Aloe Vera, coconut oil, essential oils, and honey, these are all excellent natural products for the skin. Acceding to historians, many great beauties of the past, Queen Cleopatra of Egypt being top of the list, made extensive use of honey to maintain an amazing complexion.

How Do You Keep Your Body Active?

Nothing, not even highly damaging free radicals ages the body faster than inactivity. Nature created the body to move, so restricting your movements goes against every natural law possible. The chief cause of cardiovascular problems and premature aging is inactivity. Inactivity will lead to stiff joints, flabbiness, and muscle weakness – basically, your body will waste away very quickly, your skin will go dull as an initial warning.

Stay active to keeps looking young. Exercise is a sure way of keeping your joints naturally lubricated, support body detoxification, improve lean muscle mass, increase motor functions, and build your cardiovascular health.

Congratulations! You've just discovered some important health tips which have highlighted honey as an amazing substance with powerful anti-aging properties. Honey is easy to find; easier to preserve; comes in so many different flavors and profiles; has loads of vitamins, minerals, and enzymes that boosts good health, and don't forget, it tastes so good! Honey is already being used in many traditions to create all kinds of skin care recipes (remedies) and, as pointed out just above, it can even be incorporated (or added) into the cosmetic products you are already using, this will boost results tremendously. Honey is one of the natural skin care product I use, mixed in with some perfumed cosmetic creams, and my skin actually looks better and smoother than it did in my youth. A whole chapter is dedicated to honey in this book. Read it carefully and then give honey a try. Consumed orally or rubbed on the skin, it's really an excellent anti-ager!

9. ANITOCIDANTS, ANTI-AGING, AND THE BODY

The two major causes of aging in the human body are **Oxidation** and **Free radicals**. As you get older, your body tissues suffer from oxidation due to all that oxygen you breathe in, leading to cellular damage and increased signs of aging. Free radicals are simply active chemicals that get into the body from the polluted air and environment, leading equally to cellular damage and increased signs of aging. Thrown in together, free radicals and the Oxidation process wreak havoc on body cells and this trigger accelerated aging on a grand scale. This is one major reason why people who live in cities where pollution is a major problem, and regularly get exposed to the environment, tend to look much older than normal. If you do not understand what I mean, go take a good look at the faces of footballers or sportsmen who ply their trade in open fields within polluted cities – though physically fit and youthful in body, their faces which is regularly exposed to the environment tend to look older than normal.

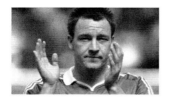

John Terry,32, Chelsea Football Cub of England…. (looks 40 at least)

A reduction in the free radical count and oxidation levels of the body will slow down aging remarkably while a hike can increase it. Antioxidants are the only compounds that attack free radicals in the body and actively counter the oxidation process at the same time! This makes all foods that have high concentrations of antioxidants superb anti-aging foods. The two, anti-aging and antioxidants go together.

10. ELEVEN TOP ANTI-AGING FOODS AND WHAT THEY OFFER

Do you want to age slower? Look a lot younger? If yes, then there are some very special nutrients you must be getting in your meals daily including antioxidants, minerals, vitamins, healthy 'good for you' fats, and phytonutrients.

Improving your diet with the careful addition of certain organic foods (fruits and vegetables) rich with these nutrients is the key: consider organic foods that have a huge positive impact on the different fundamental processes of aging in the body. And guess what? These foods can also be very delicious. You will never believe how good fighting aging can taste until you give it try!

1. Tomatoes

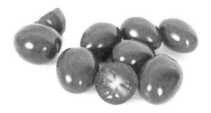

Tomatoes, a fruit originally native to South America until the conquering Spaniards brought it across the Atlantic to Europe in the 1500s, is best eaten raw (try as salad topping) but can be roasted or cooked. These delightful fruits deserve a number one position here as they are packed full of antioxidants, vitamins, and other very important nutrients (something most people are not even aware of) – vitamin C, lycopene, biotin, molybdenum, vitamin A (in the form of beta-carotene), and even vitamin K. Tomatoes are perfectly rich sources of potassium, copper, phosphorus, manganese, dietary fiber, folate, niacin, vitamin B6 and vitamin E.

These wonderful red fruits are outstanding in their high antioxidant content and richness in lycopene, both of which are very important for healthy bones, heart, blood, and skin.

These unique properties of tomatoes, all combined, have a very marked effect on the aging process of the human body. For example, the antioxidants present in tomatoes, among several other functions, fights the effects of aging brought on by the sun's harmful ultraviolet rays. How? It helps build collagen which makes your skin look healthy and youthful, even as it shields that skin from the damaging effects of the sun. Lycopene, one of the most powerful anti-aging substances known, is at the heart of the tomato. It has powerful antioxidant properties which improve the vascular system, eliminating the problem of wrinkles on your skin as well as that of a bad heart. Tomatoes improve your body's disease-fighting abilities by boosting the immune system in unique ways that cut out the possibility of heart disease and other related problems by lowering total cholesterol, low-density lipoprotein (LDL), and triglycerides, thereby leaving you with a strong heart that will function quite perfectly even as you age (this is one reason elderly people may freely engage in rigorous physical exercise even after age 70 – refer to image on book cover). In addition to its powerful antioxidant properties, tomatoes have strong anti-inflammatory properties that protects against all sorts of cancers (particularly prostate cancer), the number one disease that comes with (and accelerates) the process of aging in human beings.

Tomatoes are an amazing treasure of riches health-wise and so eating them very regularly, particularly in the raw form, will make your body healthy and highly resistant to those diseases and illnesses that accelerate aging. Eat tomatoes regularly for just six weeks and you will look and feel noticeably healthier and younger.

2. Onions

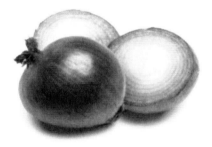

Two of the important areas this food impacts the aging process the most, and so quickly too, are in virility (the male sex drive) and eyesight, both of which wear down with age It is amazing how ignorant people are of this and all the other health benefits of onions.

Indeed, even the anti-aging benefits of this wonderful vegetable are massive, to say the least, but why health experts do not advocate it strongly is very baffling. The single compound that makes onions outstanding as a world-class anti-aging vegetable is Phytochemicals, and this is one of the best keep secrets in nutrition. The more pungent (strong) the onion – the more the antioxidant power, and this is the reason why knowledgeable people opt for white onions – it is the most powerful kind. The sulfur-rich phytochemicals, that's it! That's what gives onions their unique odor and anti-aging benefits.

One of the most powerful antioxidants known is quercetin and onions is so rich in it that no other vegetable is mentioned when speaking of this substance. Quercetin is one of the best antioxidants in the business of keeping the skin completely free of wrinkles – making a person look much younger.

Thrown in together, the sulfur-rich phytochemicals, the unique nutrients, and vitamins found abundantly in onions make it a unique vegetable best described as an anti-aging weapon, one of the best and most powerful. Onions are, indeed, very good for the skin; it protects the skin superbly, keeping it fresh (youthful looking) and smooth.

One sign of youthfulness is a full head of hair. Applied directly, onion juice stimulates hair growth; it even goes a long way in stopping hair loss, both of which becomes a huge problem with aging.

In the case of boosting male virility, onions are simply great. Onions fights impotence and weak erection in men, boosting their sex drives and confidence tremendously. The white onions are the best equipped variety for this job. Strategic but regular consumption of white onions will have a marked impact on the sex life of any man at any age. White onions, eaten raw in diets, such as salads, works wonders. One trick I frequently play on my ever-busy businessman lover is to prepare especially delicious meals for him that are heavily packed with white onions. Of course, I don't tell him a thing, but in less than one hour, he's helplessly battling a roaring erection and I become the center of his universe for quite a few days! For men with pronounced erectile dysfunction problems, give white onions soup a try, take one spoonful of honey before or after the meal, and then relax. Do this once a day for seven days and even before the period is over, you will see the changes. You can even make dense onion soup (cook 4 or 5 bulbs of onions in a pot with some water) and put it in a bottle with some honey – shake to mix. Take a small drink of it in the morning and another in the evening for 7 days. If your problem is not solved quickly by this remedy, then there is more to it than meets the eye.

The richness of onions is grossly under-rated in regards to being a source for beta-carotene, cysteine, potassium, calcium, folate and fiber. Interestingly, the total polyphenol content of onions is actually higher than in carrots, garlic, leeks, red bell pepper, and tomatoes. Yes, this means that carrots are good for your eyes but onions are much better! The best news of all is that, unlike other foods, most of the unique nutrients present in this bulb-like vegetable are not damaged when it is cooked (used in soups as described above).

Onions are not exactly the sweetest smelling of vegetables, but they will sure slow down the aging process in your body and preserve your youthful look from the inside out. They will preserve your good eyesight too. So, it's time to improve your diet with some crisp and pungent slices of onions. Try it in salads, soups, stews and side dishes.

If you ever develop the problem of sore eyes, rather than reach for some expensive synthetic eyedrop, just eat a few slices of raw onions. The effect is so fast and powerful that you will feel it even as you slice up the onions! Do not be bothered by that stinging effect which causes your eyes to water, the onions is fixing your eyes!

3. Berries

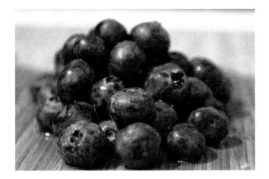

From all the many verities of berries, blueberries and raspberries stand out a mile. They are both rich in flavonoids, vitamins, polyphenols, probiotics, and tons upon tons of antioxidants, but blueberries are something more. Blueberries are a super fruit that helps counter the physical and mental effects of the aging process.

Thanks to their amazing richness in antioxidants, these tiny blue fruits called blueberries help clean up the free radicals and toxins in your body which are associated with diseases and aging. Blueberries are truly a gift of nature to the betterment of human health, but despite being so rich in medicinal nutrients, they still taste so wonderful. Blueberries have the highest concentration of antioxidants among all the berries – strawberries, raspberries, blackberries – it beats them all. In additions, there are certain compounds percent in blueberries which prevent cells in the human body from aging, this helps you look and feel younger and it even improves your mental capacity as well.

The strong color of blueberries is due to its richness in anthocyanin, a substance with powerful anti-inflammatory properties which slows down the ugly process of loss of mental function with aging – this is one reason blueberries are just about the only fruits known to slow down the cognitive deterioration of the brain which comes with Alzheimer's disease.

A lot of other age-related problems such as loss of orientation, fitness, and sense of organization, all of which are major factors in age-related accidents, are brought under control by compounds present in blueberries. There are even known cases where a person's motor function skills improve rapidly with regular consumption of blueberries.

Although blueberries are so sweet, they are remarkably low on calories and sugar (Blueberries are in the category of glycemic index foods which means your blood sugar won't go high when you eat them a lot, this means zero worries about diabetes! Unlike other fruits, blueberries are packed with nutrients and all kinds of compounds –

tannins, flavonoids, iron, manganese, Vitamin C and E, antioxidants and phytochemicals – which prevent chronic illnesses and deadly diseases like cancer, diabetes and heart disease. How? The simple answer is that all these special compounds combine to protect our DNA in unique ways that keep us very healthy. Blueberries also lower cholesterol levels and improve the eyesight at the same time.

With the problem of halting skin aging and preventing wrinkles, blueberries, with its powerful anti-inflammatory properties is simply wonderful! Are you suffering from an age-related sickness like arthritis or cancer? This high anti-inflammatory property of Blueberries is just for you. But if you had added this amazing fruit to your diet early enough, arthritis and cancer never would have taken root in your body in the first place!

To keep looking healthy and younger, eat blueberries regularly. These free-radical scavengers will protect you adequately from all manner of polluted environment — from air pollution that damages your skin and pumps harmful chemicals into your body to water pollution that harms you directly from the inside out. Blueberries even promote cell regeneration, ensuring you have new and youthful looking skin at all times.

51

4. Green Tea

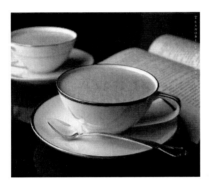

Green tea, which is native to the Orient, comes in with the complex activity of fighting aging at cellular level. It helps with correct cellular regeneration which keeps you looking and feeling very young for as long as possible. Since cell mutation can lead to anything from uneven pigmentation to cancer, green tea is very important for our health. Green tea is rich in antioxidants as well as a chemical called EGCG which help all body cells grow perfectly and maintain a healthy life cycle.

The Japanese and the Chines have used green tea for a thousand years as a defense against aging. The Japanese, who tend to live for so long, credit green tea for the lengthy lifespan. Japanese scientists say Green tea even helps with weight loss and that's true because it's got all the right compounds in rich supply, even beneficial acids, which act as antioxidants.

According to a study carried out by some Chinese experts, men who consumed green tea regularly had their cells aging at a much slower rate than those who didn't. The unique antioxidants percent in Green tea are responsible for this phenomenon.

Middle-aged and elderly folk will sure be delighted to learn that Green tea contains powerful flavonoids that act as lubricants to the joints, particularly the knees. In a unique manner, Green tea reduces collagen and cartilage destruction in arthritic joints, and this helps in the prevention and control of both osteoarthritis and rheumatoid arthritis.

Green tea has the highest known concentrations of polyphenols and catechins, both powerful antioxidants which do battle with all manner of free radicals in your body to maintain your vibrant and youthful look. These unique antioxidant properties also make Green tea a superb moisturizer when applied directly to the skin. It can cleanse the skin deeply and make it radiant in little time – a ball of cotton wool and the remaining part of a cup of Green tea are all you need. Soak up the tea with the cotton wool and apply directly to your skin.

Green tea also contains high levels of yet another one of the most potent antioxidant known to medicine – oligomeric proanthocyanins (OPCs). Researchers have proven that this substance practically slows down premature aging if consumed orally (internally). Whether the case is the same when Green tea is applied directly on the skin (externally) is yet to be proven, though so many believe it does.

So now you know about this super healthy beverage, it's time for a switch. Green tea will make you several years younger even as it increases your lifespan.

5. Kefir and Yogurt

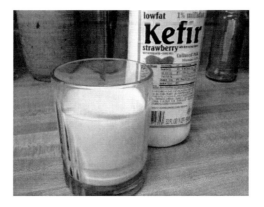

We all know what yogurt is and have even tasted it at one time or another, but what is Kefir?

Kefir is much like yogurt, a sour-sweet drink made from the fermentation process of the dairy product, milk. Strangely enough, both end up becoming far more nutritious than milk, but Kefir stands out a mile. Milk is good for your health but yogurt is far much better while Kefir puts yogurt to shame seven times over!

Fondly called the Champagne of milk due to an effervescence which makes it bubbly, Kafir is originally from the northern region of the Caucasus Mountains (the highest section of the Alps mountain range dividing Europe from Asia). Kefir is made by heating milk, to kill off any unwanted bacteria, and then adding a special yeast and bacteria mix, which begins the fermentation process. The end product is a substance so rich in nutrients and living probiotics (body friendly bacteria), its health benefits are off the charts. The people of the Caucasus Mountains have been drinking kefir daily for a thousand years and are said to live very long and healthy lives indeed. The crisp and clean mountain air can't be held responsible for this unusual longevity but kefir's massive health and anti-aging benefits, as seen below, definitely can.

Kefir is a rich and natural source of the vitamin B complex which are very important for the maintenance of proper body functions – healthy skin, a healthy nervous system and healthy digestive system. Its anti-stress properties help immensely with the nervous system. Kefir contains a good supply of tryptophan, an amino acid which is one of the essential building blocks required by the body to produce proteins, replace cells and maintain a healthy nervous system.

Kefir is literally trillions of body friendly micro-organisms in one cup! Called probiotics, these bacteria do your body a world of good from the inside out. In that single cup of kefir, you get about 3 trillion good micro-organisms; so many tiny, little 'bugs' that work wonders in your body all in one drink!

Yet another health benefit of kefir is better metabolism. Drinking Kefir as an after-meal treat will improve your digestive system and regulate bowel movements. This property might not line up as one that explains the long lives of kefir-drinking people, however, it is a useful health practice which will definitely lead to other benefits in your body.

Cholesterol comes in two divisions: good cholesterol and bad cholesterol. The bad cholesterol, known as Low-density lipoprotein (LDL) is responsible for the clogging up of arteries, which cause cardiovascular problems such as heart attacks and strokes. Kefir is one food that will actively reduce the LDL cholesterol levels in your blood, thereby keeping your heart healthy.

For the millions of people who have allergies or digestive problems relating to milk and the lactose in it, kefir is a welcome diet. The fermentation process of the milk into kefir keeps all the good properties but gets rid of the problematic one: the lactose is converted into lactic acid while all the vitamins and minerals are preserved.

The anti-aging and life-prolonging benefits of Kefir are in no doubt as both the people of the Caucasus Mountains and several renowned scientists have held the view for hundreds of years. In fact, over one hundred years ago, the renowned Nobel prize winning scientist, Elie Metchnikoff, conducted numerous research on the subject and published many papers on it.

Among many things, Kefir fortifies the body's immune system greatly and speeds up healing processes. Thanks to its powerful antibacterial, antiviral and antifungal properties, which help ward off diseases and fight infections, even regular ailments like colds and coughs never take hold in the body.

Kefir's richness in antioxidants is another reason for its lofty reputation as an anti-aging food. Drinking Kefir regularly helps with body detoxification which slows down the process of aging and keeps you looking younger for longer.

Lastly, Kefir, being a rich source of important vitamins and minerals, can boost your energy levels tremendously, and herein lies buried another secret: Kefir boasts both male virility and the human sex drive! The presence of calcium and magnesium in Kefir guarantees strong bones and teeth while the vitamins A, B complex and K, help with everything from good eyesight to good skin. Throw in all those healthy probiotics and it's all too good to be true!

To stay happy and healthy, you sure need foods like Kefir. You'll find it in the dairy sections of most supermarkets where it's often sold as a beverage.

6. Fish

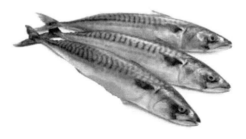

Fish oils are very high in omega-3 fatty acids, which is one of the best fats for your body. We are not just talking just any fish here, though, but a particular group of oily fishes which have their home mostly in the Atlantic Ocean.

The health benefits of fish oils are simply endless. In addition to strengthening the heart, brain, skin and overall body health, fish oils prevent cancer, eye diseases, and bone problems. Yes, indeed, the health benefits of fish oils are almost without end but only recently did a new study link it directly to the prevention of premature aging and this is why '**fish**' is on our list of important anti-aging foods.

First class omega-3 oils can only be gotten through a healthy diet of the right fishes, and since they are polyunsaturated fats, which is a **'very healthy'** fat unlike saturated animal fats – they don't raise your cholesterol levels but help in lowering it instead. Yes, fish oils improve your health and aid weight loss.

Polyunsaturated fats are split into two groups under Essential Fatty Acids (EFAs) - omega-3 and omega-6. Both groups are essential in the regulation of body temperature, blood clotting, blood pressure and the immune system. They are also required in the production of prostaglandins, which are very important hormone-like chemicals present in the body.

Omega-3 is particularly beneficial in the production of essential substances like DHA (docosahexaenoic acid), which plays a vital role in the development of the brain and reasoning functions. It also contributes to the production of Eicosapentaenoic acid (EPA), yet another important compound required for optimal brain health.

Fish oils are actually the richest sources of omega-3s but – as pointed out earlier – not just any fish. The following are the fishes you want to eat – salmon, Atlantic mackerel, fresh tuna, and herring. Wild salmon, in particular, is incredible when you want to have beautiful and younger looking skin. Most edible oils and other foods – corn and sunflower oils, even red meat – will give you good supplies of omega-6 but are deficient in omega-3.

According to a study published in the Journal of The American College of Cardiology, fish oils will boost your brain health tremendously. The study which was directed by Dr. Carl Lavie, of the prestigious Ochsner Cardiology Clinic in Louisiana, USA, also showed that omega-3 fatty oils help to prevent blood clotting and regulate blood pressure (lowered it). Clearly, fish oils have powerful heart-protection abilities that elderly people with established cardiovascular diseases will find lifesaving. Elderly people with Alzheimer's disease are not left out; they are helped greatly by the brain power boosting effects of fish oils, thanks to DHA which cuts down the formation of plaques in the brain.

Of note here is that though DHA has been shown to boost brain development on major levels. it does not boost intelligence. So parents who pump their children full of fish oil capsules (or other related supplements) ahead of big exams are basically throwing away their money, or not quite, just adding more vitamin A and E to the child's system the expensive way is more like it!

Fish oils are superb in regards to anti-aging. Researchers from the University of California have found that omega-3 rich foods and supplements help greatly in cell regeneration and protection, which in turn, leads to better protection against inflammation and the entire aging process. Basically, the more omega-3 (or fish oil) you consume, the slower the damage to the DNA in your cells.

So, will fish oil effectively make you look younger? The answer – based on the physical evidence of very healthy people who eat fish day in, day out, in countries like Japan – is yes! Interestingly, though, some experts will tell you that more research is required on the subject. What these experts really mean is that they want to spend more funds and get the facts down on paper in their private labs so as to take all the credit despite clear evidence already staring them in the eyes.

For over a thousand years, the fish-eating Japanese have lived very healthy, very active and very long lives. Some traditional Japanese Samurai fighters of ancient times lived to well over 80 years of age before retirement just on diets of fish and seaweed.

Eating oily fish diets at least once a week will not just make you look younger but will protect you completely against age-related diseases like macular degeneration, the number one cause of blindness in older people. Fish oil also do battle with some forms of cancer – it cuts out the possibility of prostate cancer and bowel cancer completely.

The best sources of omega-3 are fish oils, and this is best gotten by the consumption of the right oily fishes – salmon, mackerel, fresh tuna, etc. Fish oil pills are not quite right and other sources of omega-3 are even less a match. These other sources of omega-3 include, walnut oils, rapeseed, and evening primrose, fresh seeds such as sunflower and pumpkin, whole-grain bread and wholegrain cereals like wheat and soybeans – they all provide omega-3s in a different chemical form which the body cannot absorb readily and convert into DHA and EPA. This means that going by alternative sources, you will never get enough omega-3 compounds in your system.

As a doctor, my recommendation for good health in certain conditions where the right oily fishes can't be gotten and consumed is to take 500mg of omega-3 fish oil capsules each day. Where the patient suffers from heart failure or heart disease, I recommend at least 800 to 1000mg to go with their daily diet. However, I always say this, "If you made it a habit of eating just one whole mackerel fish a week, none of this would have happened in the first place."

Note – It is infinitely better to eat the fish to provide the oil than to take the pill. In addition to the right chemical compounds, you also get a ton of other important nutrients and proteins by eating the fish– many a medical expert will tell you this same thing. Suggestions to take supplements instead of the fish itself remains controversial, the world over.

Have you suffered a heart attack? Fish dosage: Eat two to three portions of oily fish a week. DO NOT TAKE FISH OIL CAPSULES.

Do you want to look younger and feel healthier? Fish dosage: One to two portions of oily fish a week. DO NOT RELY ON CAPSULES.

The most popular fish oil capsule, Cod liver oil actually contains some EPA and DHA, but in inferior quantities compared to any of the oily fishes. Unlike other capsules, cod liver oil contains vitamin D, an important vitamin which is absent in people who live in countries where getting regular sunlight is a problem (the action of sunlight on the skin is the main source of this important vitamin). A deficiency in Vitamin D is directly linked to a whole range of health complications and diabetes is top of the pack, followed by bone disease and even rickets, which is making a name for itself in the United Kingdom.

Are you living in a country where regular sunlight is a major problem and don't eat the right fishes? Take a regular dosage of cod liver oil and do not forget to give some to your kids.

7. Nuts

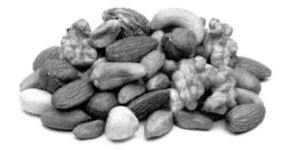

Do you wish to live long? Go nuts today! The New England Journal of Medicine says you can live for up to 80 or 90 years in superb health by just eating a handful of nuts daily!

From Europe to the United States, renowned medical experts have carried out so much research on nuts as relating to longevity. Although they agree that people who eat a handful of mixed nuts on a daily basis have a very little risk of ever developing cancer, heart diseases, and other age-related ailments, the number one nut that stands out of the pack is **walnut**.

Walnuts, though somewhat dry, have a massive impact on health and longevity. Almonds, peanuts, Brazilian nuts, pine nuts, and pistachios, are all superb for perfect health and long life too, but this is not to say you should go over feeding on them. A handful of nuts a day will do just fine as pointed out above. Let's take a look at some of the health benefits of eating these nuts regularly.

Walnuts are very rich in the rare omega-3 fatty acids that are found only in certain fish. These fatty acids, in conjunction with other vital nutrients and minerals present in the nut, make it so important for good health and longevity. Studies have made it clearly known that walnuts fight all kinds of cancer and improves brain power (boosts memory, improves concentration and information processing speed), reduces the risks of diabetes, reduces inflammation and promotes dilated and relaxed blood vessels, which in turn sets back the time on heart disease, and, incredibly, boosts male fertility markedly. According to the Walnuts and Healthy Aging (WAHA), daily consumption of walnut positively influences blood cholesterol levels without any negative effects on body weight in older adults. Another benefit of eating the walnut daily is that it alters the bacteria present in the stomach in a way that decreases inflammation and cholesterol levels in the entire body (note – inflammation and cholesterol levels are two known indicators of heart health). Want to stop eating too much, slim down and look younger? Acceding to research from the University of Georgia, USA, eating a diet rich in polyunsaturated fat after meals that are high in saturated fat (which makes you fat), favorably modifies hunger and satisfaction levels in the body. Simply put, you eat less and less but always get satisfied. Walnuts are indeed a great source for polyunsaturated fat.

Peanuts (or groundnuts as it's called in some lands) are an anti-aging sludge hammer and they are so tasty too! In the class, legumes, peanuts are very rich in the potent antioxidant called resveratrol (a substance found in dark chocolate and red wine). Resveratrol slows aging markedly and reduces the risk of cardiovascular (heart) disease. Peanuts improve brain health too, thanks to their high vitamin E and folic acid content. Niacin, folate, protein and manganese are the other important substances you can get from peanuts as your regular butter.

Brazil Nuts are a powerhouse nutritionally. They are rich in selenium, a substance required by the body in the production of illness-fighting antioxidants. Then there's the zinc too.

As you age, your skin becomes more delicate and this is where Zinc comes in, particularly if you are prone to cuts at your workplace. Zinc fixes the problem by helping with new skin production. Brazil nuts are very rich in zinc and so you will need them a lot. Prostate cancer is another reason why you need Brazil nuts, it potentially eliminates the possibility of this disease.

Almonds contain, to some degree, all the nutritional benefits of their kin, but the rich amount of healthy vegetable protein they have to offer is the highest of the pack. They are also very rich in calcium, which is needed for bones health, and vitamin E, which boosts memory and reduce mental decline.

Pine Nuts can lower bad LDL cholesterol significantly. It is rich in manganese, which is an essential component in the formation of one of the body's most powerful antioxidants.

Pistachios are superb in the boosting of arterial health. Its l-arginine content makes the lining of the arteries more flexible, and in turn, this potentially reduces the risks of heart attack and stroke. Pistachios are lower in calories which tell a lot about your weight issues.

Aside from these nuts mentioned above, all others are unimportant in their impact on anti-aging and perfect health. In regards to health benefits, in particular, these other nuts merely replicate the nutrients present in the nuts mentioned above but to a lesser degree.

8. Avocados

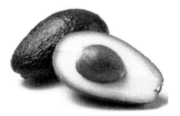

Avocados, like fish and nuts, are rich in important fats and nutrient, but that's not all. Avocados also have lots of glutathione, another powerful anti-aging substance. Glutathione is wonderful for detoxing the body. What I mean is this; glutathione flushes out toxins from your system, thereby keeping acne and wrinkles at bay.

For several decades, avocados were categorized as fatty food and avoided, but new findings have revealed that all that fat is monounsaturated, and this puts avocado in the class of fish – foods full of fats that are simply good for you. Avocado even protects against heart disease and certain cancers.

With the discovery of the health benefits of its monounsaturated fats content, the popularity of avocados has skyrocketed. Avocados actually lowers cholesterol levels, not raise them as previously thought. In fact, nutritionally, avocados are perfect balanced. Avocados contain almost all the important nutrients that the bodies cannot produce on its own or do without. What about looking younger? Avocados offer an incredible number of antioxidants that can turn back the time on aging (reverse aging).

Most people are ignorant of the powerful anti-aging properties contained in both the oil and the flesh of avocados. Avocados contain potent anti-aging properties that protect the body against free radicals. Interestingly, research has shown that Avocados have the ability to penetrate deeply into the body's cell structures, entering the mitochondria and activating its energy production so the cells function properly even under constant attack by free radicals. The mitochondria are central mechanisms of cells, and there, are the bulk of the cell's energy produced using nutrients. Mitochondria plays a very vital role in the body's endless fight against free radicals which accelerate aging. However, there is a side effect – mitochondria generate unstable chemicals that damage both the mitochondrial mechanism themselves and other cellular mechanisms. This damage has a negative impact on aging which many scientists worked tirelessly to reverse. They have found an adequate solution in avocado oil!

Avocado oil causes accelerated respiration in the mitochondria, which guarantees that all required cell functions are highly effective even in cells attacked by free radicals, but the production of those damaging chemicals are cut back.

Avocados contain about 20 vital nutrients which include: Calcium, Fiber, Potassium (over twice the amount found in a banana), Vitamin A, vitamin E, Vitamin D, the

B-complex vitamins, Iron, Sodium, Magnesium, Folic acid, and Boron. But that isn't all, avocados increase the body's ability to absorb fat-soluble nutrients from other vegetables and fruits such as alpha, beta-carotene, and lutein. The antibacterial, antiviral and antifungal properties of avocado boost the immune system impressively. Avocados' richness in the amino acid known as lecithin, guarantees that illnesses like liver overload, will never be a problem; it also helps in balancing body weight, rejuvenates the skin and boosts brain functions immensely.

Avocado also boosts the production of collagen which helps prevent the effects of aging on the skin. It also helps with bad sight, thanks to a rich supply of vitamin A. The health benefits of this fruit are simply endless. Perhaps you should give it a try today.

9. Honey

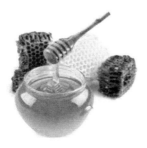

Do you have a sweet tooth? Substitute honey for sugar in your diet to stay healthy and youthful. The health and anti-aging benefits of honey have been drummed about for thousands of years but only recently did modern scientists really figure out why. In addition to its powerful antiviral, antifungal, and antibacterial properties, honey is packed full of antioxidants. It is even an antioxidant all by itself! Incredible is the fact that, though technically sugar, honey doesn't cause inflammation in the body and skin like regular sugar does but has a positive impact instead.

We will dwell more on honey later.

10. Cucumbers

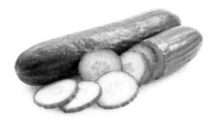

Just one cucumber a day takes the age away! Yes, cucumber has the ability to knock decades off your life if you use it just right.

Historians report that Cleopatra, the mightiest queen of ancient Egypt, consumed cucumber salads and used milk and honey on her skin to remain a very youthful and glowing beauty all her life. Little wonder the greatest general of Rome, Mark Antony, fell helplessly at her feet!

A few years ago, I had the pleasure of getting to know a lovely lady during a dinner in one of the larger West African countries I once visited on charity work. She looked no more than 30 and so I nearly had a heart attack when I learned she was actually 48. Her secret – cucumbers and honey, with lots and lots of water! Chief Mrs. Benson, drinks cups of water for lunch daily, eats one cucumber salad each morning and used honey on her face at least once a week. That's about it.

Like honey, cucumbers have massive anti-inflammatory and anti-aging properties. They are so rich in vitamin A, vitamin K, potassium, and silica, all of which are needed to strengthen the connective tissues that hold the organs and muscles in the body together. Now, there you have the explanation: why you get to look so young with one cucumber a day!

Cucumber, being rich in vitamin A, is excellent for the eyes. Squeeze some drops of cucumber juice into your eyes at night, before you go to sleep. Do this at least once a week. Another trick is to relax with slices of cucumber over the eyes for a while.

11. Olive oil

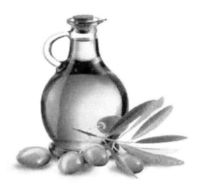

Olive oil is a product of the fruits harvested from olive trees. Its popularity is due to its immense health benefits and culinary usefulness. Olive oil is used in numerous diet plans due to its richness in monounsaturated fatty acids, which promotes good health and weight loss. It also boosts heart health, regulates high blood pressure and cuts down the risk of heart attack and stroke. Due to its unique richness in vitamin E, a powerful anti-oxidant known for its anti-aging properties, olive oil has a lot of impact on the eyes, skin, and overall neurological health. Alternatively, olive oil is used in cooking, but it's also super when used to nurture hair and skin.

The origin of olive oil is dealt with in the section for essential oils which is to come.

11. OTHER VITAL ANTI-AGING FOODS AND DELICIOUS WAYS TO EAT THEM

As pointed out earlier, one of the most effective ways to halt the unwelcome natural process of aging in the body is by preparing and enjoying particular foods. And they can be quite delicious too!

1. Pomegranates

Packed with vitamin C, ellagic acid, and punicalagin, permanganate is one fruit that keeps you looking younger by guarding your skin against the damaging effects of the sun and getting rid of wrinkles. The juice gotten from pomegranate seeds is rich in ellagic acid and punicalagin:

Ellagic acid is a powerful polyphenol compound that helps the body fight damage from toxins and free radicals while punicalagin is a super-nutrient that heightens your body's ability to preserve collagen (that subdermal connective tissue that helps the skin look smooth and youthful.

A few of these lovely red juicy permanganate fruits, eaten wholly on a weekly basis, will do you so much good.

2. Garlic

Garlic is the herb legend claims keeps vampires away, but it actually does a lot better than that by keeping you from joining the same vampires in a coffin!

This herb, with its rich and strong flavor, slows down the aging process remarkably and prolongs your life. Garlic has a wide variety of healing properties as well as powerful antibacterial, antiviral, and antifungal properties, all of which have been well known and well used in many traditions and civilizations for hundreds of years. Garlic, in addition to being an immune system booster, prevents colds, removes warts, and even helps treat athlete's foot.

With its high bacteria, virus, and fungus fighting properties, coupled with a richness in Sulphur, garlic is a very potent anti-aging food that's wonderful for the health of the skin and liver. It boosts the cardiovascular system (cutting down heart diseases markedly), regulates blood pressure (which helps the heart and brain) and lowers cholesterol levels (which checks weight gain and heart diseases).

Feel free to add Garlic to your diet at least twice or thrice a week but no more because the chemicals responsible for its pungent flavor have the ability to alter your body's natural scent if consumed too much – people who have the habit of eating several raw bulbs of garlic daily (such as the Koreans and some Indians), smell strongly of the herb in a way a lot of other people find repulsive. A safe, delicious and 'easy to prepare' recipe to try is Garlic Chicken, which you can't eat more than once or twice a week anyway. Since garlic comes in the powdered form (as cooking spice), a few shots in water is another fantastic way to add this herb to your diet.

3. Fiber-Rich Grains

In addition to having marked anti-aging properties, fiber-rich grains have several health benefits, which include weight loss, better heart health, and lower blood sugar. They basically soak up most of the bad substances in your body and take them out.

4. Leafy Green Vegetables

Pumpkin, broccoli, kale, turnip greens, spinach, cabbage, and even edible seaweed – packed with vitamins, minerals and nutrients, these green leafy vegetables all have the power to induce good health but they also slow down the aging process to a crawl. In addition, these wonderful vegetables are very rich in fiber, meaning they can sweep your system clean of harmful substances. Seaweed is by far the richest and most nourishing vegetable known. Seaweed contains almost every important nutrient and vitamin you can think of, and then some more. It even contains iodine and soda, two of the rarest chemicals to come by in vegetables and fruits. The Japanese who live extraordinarily long lives, by tradition, eat richly of fresh seaweed with almost every meal as they have been doing for a thousand years.

Sea wrecked sailors in the vast Pacific Ocean have been known to survive and even live very healthy lives on desolate islands for months just by feeding on fresh seaweed alone! The only disadvantage being that they often have greenish skin as a result of its high Chlorophyll content (the Indian verity of spinach has this problem too but is so tasty that African's don't mind squeezing out the leaves several times over with hot water to get rid of the Chlorophyll before adding to soups or stews).

Pumpkin, particularly the West African variety, is another green leafy vegetable so rich in nutrients, proteins, and vitamins, it can give you a healthy life all by itself if eaten regularly as food alone (as in vegetarian diets).

Watercress

This ordinary looking vegetable are mentioned separately because of their exceptional nature that pushes them slightly outside the circle of green leafy vegetables, making them one of the most powerful anti-aging foods known to man.

The US Centers for Disease Control and Prevention have watercress ranked as highest among the vegetables in terms of nutrient density. The experts down there at the CDCP actually place Watercress well above spinach, cabbages, kale, and swiss chard. This is a bit difficult to believe, particularly for a person like me who has seen what these and other green vegetables can do. Take seaweed and pumpkin, for example, the things these vegetables do for the long-living Japanese and super healthy West African tribes respectively, are best described as wonders.

The only area where watercress has an upper hand over other green leafy vegetables is in its rich sulfur content which gives it unique similarities to onions and garlic.

Sulfur is outstanding for good health and so is Watercress. Replace the cabbage and spinach in your diets with some tasty green Watercress today!

Eating these amazing green leafy vegetables, all fresh and raw, is the perfect way to get the best of everything out of them. A delicious spicy vegetable Salad is just one of many good ways to add them to your food on a daily basis.

5. Red Wine

Now we are talking!

For about two thousand years, human beings have drunk richly of red wine without a hint of its amazing anti-aging properties even though it stared them right in the eyes, day after day, with the evidence of people living very long and healthy lives. Indeed, it was only just recently that scientific research confirmed the suspicion of many health experts; that red wine possessed multiple health benefits which included anti-aging properties. Red wine contains an important antioxidant known as resveratrol which counters the aging process. The wine is known to reduce bad cholesterol and increase lifespan. How exactly it does the latter is not well known yet, but hey! Let that not stop you from having a glass of red wine with one of your meals daily. There are many varieties of red wine to choose from so there is sure to be one that will please you.

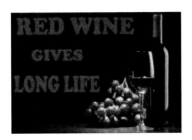

Warning: Red wine contains more calories than most other alcoholic beverages including beers and spirits. In addition to this, its resveratrol content is not that high too. Another worrying point is its alcohol content. The body simply does not do well with lots of alcohol in it and so if you go drowning bottles of upon bottles of red wine in your desire to live long, all you'll get is very fat and full of illnesses very quickly.

Anything over two glasses of red wine a day is too much.

6. Legumes

Beans are highly beneficial in the body's endless fight against aging. Being high in fiber, Beans are known to lower cholesterol, and blood sugar levels, help beneficial bacteria grow in the gut and supply the body with all kinds of vital nutrients and vitamins. Beans are one of the easiest foods to prepare and some ingredients that go with it in some lands, such as potash alum, makes it a powerful cancer prevention and fighting weapon. Don't skip the chance to enjoy some delicious and healthy Bean Salad meal at least once a week.

7. Cruciferous Vegetables

Brussels sprouts, Turnips, and radishes are all powerful anti-aging vegetables. They have rich nutritional content that strengthens the body's ability to remain healthy and fight off diseases. They also have high antioxidant content that protects the skin and the body against rampaging free radicals which cause faster aging. Like all vegetables go, it is advisable to eat these ones raw for best results but they often retain enough nutrients when cooked. Roasting tastes better, so give Roasted Turnips with Ginger a try and thank me later.

8. Ginger

Ginger is a delicious spice with massive health and anti-aging properties that have made it the darling of Asian ladies for hundreds of years. Apart from being packed with nutrients, Ginger has anti-inflammatory properties that soothe arthritic symptoms. Simply put, Ginger is to the joints what lubricants are to metal hinges, metal joints, and motor engines – it keeps things in the joints well-oiled and smooth moving. Ginger is also useful in combating nausea, hangovers, and abdominal cramps (women with painful menstrual periods should try drinking ginger in **warm** water). Spice up your food with ginger or consume it as a soothing tea.

9. Salmon

Mentioned under the 'Oily Fish' topic above, Salmon has a very high antioxidant content which makes it a potent weapon in the fight against the aging process. It's high omega-3 content and other related nutrients make it extremely good for the heart, the skin and the brain. Salmon is certainly one of the best foods to start adding to your diet if you want to feel and look younger. Enjoy fried Salmon with stewed rice for added nutrition.

10. Orange Vegetables

Sweet potatoes, carrots, and squash are packed with nutrients, vitamins, and antioxidants, all of which have powerful anti-aging properties. These unique vegetables also contain high amounts of beta-carotene, an essential nutrient for good eyes. Try some Sweet Carrots in your salad today.

11. Watermelon

Watermelon, a powerful stakeholder in the anti-aging sector, is simply delicious! It has powerful disease fighting properties and aids weight loss. Try watermelon as a salad, add red onion, feta cheese, black olives, and olive oil as dressings – enjoy!

12. MORE UNIQUE FOODS FOR YOUR ANTI-AGING DIET

Antioxidant Rich Teas

Green tea has been mentioned already, however, there are other teas with lesser but still important anti-aging properties which make them worth mentioning. White tea, rooibos tea, black tea and oolong tea – there they are. These teas are all rich in a certain group of antioxidants called polyphenols, which protects body cells from the damaging attacks of free radicals.

Wild-caught fish

All wild caught oily fish in the class of the Salmon contains unique levels of Vitamin D and astaxanthins so high, they are off the charts. The fishes furnish the body with the anti-inflammatory fatty oil, omega-3, which slows down the aging process to a marked degree. The vitamins do the same thing too but all these nutrients, combined, boost brain and heart health.

Herbs

We've mentioned garlic before but another herb worth mentioning here is Turmeric. This herb is quite rich in antioxidants and deep cleansing nutrients that can particularly slow down the aging process when used right.

13. FOODS THAT CAUSE FASTER AGING IN HUMANS

If you want to avoid aging, here are the foods to avoid in your daily diet at all costs. These foods do nothing but accelerate the aging process and do major harm to the body in many other different ways.

Refined sugar

This bleached sweet substance, when consumed, promotes a certain process called glycation. Glycation is directly responsible for damaging body cells on all levels and thus, causing skin wrinkles. Sugar is the world's number one food when it comes to speeding up the aging process in the human body.

Grains

Yeah, you heard right. Grains like wheat and even corn are pro-inflammatory if not sprouted (grown) and will lead to the production of glycation in the body, and as you now know, glycation does nothing but speed up the aging process in our bodies.

Trans fats and hydrogenated oils

Stir well clear of these particularly processed fats as they are known to promote inflammation which not only leads to premature aging but certain types of cancer and heart disease as well.

Alcohol

Stop drinking alcohol already! Aside from red wine which has well-proven health benefits if taken in moderation, all the rest of the other wines are just alcohol and unhealthy chemicals with different forms of sugar. Consumed, alcohol is pro-inflammatory and speeds up the ugly aging process in a major way which begins with an increase in your waistline and then the destruction of your skin. Other effects of alcohol intake included increased risks of chronic diseases such as heart attack, stroke, diabetes, liver diseases, brain disorders, cell damage and death (particularly in younger people and women),

Artificial Sugar and Other Such Artificial Ingredients

Surely, we do not need a doctor to tell us that these substances – surgery soft drinks, processed beverages and ice-creams – are no good. Not after reading this book to this point. These substances contain a staggering number of chemicals which can speed up the aging process in style, the processed sugar that makes them so sweet is just one. Regular consumption of these processed foods gives nothing but ill-health.

14. POPULAR EVERYDAY FOODS THAT SPEED UP AGING

Fast foods are a big 'no, no' since all they offer are foods that speed up the aging process such as fries, burgers, and sugar. Almost nothing organic come out of these fast foods outlets. It's all processed foods, and processed food are loaded with chemicals which make them sweeter, not healthier.

French fries and Potato chips

Any food that is deep-fried in saturated oil does nothing but add to inflammation throughout your body. Avoid trans-fats in particular. Trans-fats have the unwelcome ability to raise your levels of "bad" cholesterol (LDL) and lower the levels of "good" cholesterol, (HDL). Basically, when you eat these tasty fries, you are increasing your risk of getting heart disease and cancer.

Check the labels on packaged baked foods and crackers, lookout for these highlights, "**partially** hydrogenated oils" and "vegetable shortening.". If found, do not eat!

Doughnuts and sugary pastries.

These snacks are packed with sugar and other processed substances which do your body a lot of harm as well as fostering the development of wrinkles.

Bacon, Hot dogs, and Pepperoni

It's a well-established fact that processed meats are very high in saturated fats, in addition to being packed with nitrates. These food lead nowhere but to inflammation and cancer.

Fatty meats.

Rich or fatty meats are loaded with saturated fats. Keeping meat lean, that's the key! Go for ground beef that is no less than 95% lean. Ground chicken and turkey breast are other fine opinions for lean meat.

15. TOP TEN ANTI-AGING SUPPLEMENTS AND WHAT THEY DO WITHIN YOU

Do you have little time for healthy food but often worry that you are aging too fast? Have you ever wished for some sort of magic pill which can slow down that troubling aging process and keep you looking younger for even longer?

We age faster than ever every day, thanks to the pollution in the environment and the type of food we consume.

So, how do we tackle this problem? Are there any anti-aging supplements that you can use? Well, there are some powerful anti-aging supplements you can use to knock back the hands of the clock on the aging process in your body! This chapter brings knowledge of these supplements right to you.

1. Omega-3 fats (Fish Oil, 1000 mg daily)

Fish oils which are rich in omega-3 fats DHA and EPA, are very powerful anti-inflammatory agents which are known to drastically reduce age-related cellular damage.

Regular consumption of Omega-3 is also a medically proficient way of keeping the heart hale and healthy.

In addition to improving eyesight markedly, Omega-3 cuts down the damaging effects of glaucoma and macular degeneration. In the case of people with heart problems, this unique supplement helps in increasing their lifespan by reducing the chances of sudden death.

2. Green superfood powder (1 scoop daily)

This substance is drawn from foods high in antioxidant compounds such as chlorella, wild berries, grass juices, and herbs, all of which slow down the aging process markedly.

3. Resveratrol (250-500 mg daily)

This substance is a polyphenol found solely in red grapes and berries. The effectiveness of this substance is frequently linked to the old idea that wine (red wine in particular) is the secret behind a long and healthy life.

Resveratrol is great news for diabetic patients as it is known to increase their insulin sensitivity by decreasing the glucose levels in their system.

In normal people, Resveratrol is noted for the maintenance of a protein called *sirtuin*, which enhances the longevity of cells. Take the recommended dosage of this supplement for a longer lifespan.

4. Adaptogen Herbs, Rhodiola, Ashwagandha, Holy Basil, Ginseng (500-1000 mg daily)

These unique herbs work by reducing cortisol levels in the system and cutting down the normal damaging effects of stress on the body in general.

5. Co-enzyme Q10 (150 mg 2x daily)

As we grow older, the body's production of a particular enzyme called CoQ10 decreases rapidly. Parkinson's disease, diabetes, and cancer – these are just a few of the diseases linked to a low production of this enzyme CoQ10 in the body.

That's not all. Numerous researchers have proven the ability of this unique enzyme, CoQ10 to promote heart functions by efficiently preventing the blood from clotting in unique ways. This helps in reducing the chances of heart attack and other heart-related diseases.

CoQ10 also acts as a powerful antioxidant and is required for energy production in body cells. It protects the cells from damage, thereby resulting in heightened overall health and a cut down in the aging process.

6. Aspirin:

This traditional pains and fever killer is actually a wonder drug that is now prescribed for various other ailments. Why? While studies have revealed that those who take small doses of this drug daily have better overall health, doctors cannot overlook the evidence anymore.

How Aspirin Work....

Aspirin simply thins out the blood which in turn leads to its better flow through the veins, and thus, greatly lessening the possibility of clotting. Better blood circulation translates to better blood flow to all body organs, which subsequently function perfectly.

Aspirin is also known to prevent colon cancer. The risk of this disease is cut back by at least 55% in those who take this drug on alternate days.

7. Carnitine:

Stored in different parts of the body, this nutrient helps in the conversion of stored fat into energy. In healthy humans, the liver and kidney produce this element but production levels decrease considerably with passing years.

People with chest pain problems should take the recommended dosage of this supplement to treat. Those with emerging signs of Alzheimer's disease also need it. This supplement helps markedly in the treatment of depression and dementia.

Incredibly enough this supplement has one other good health benefit. When taken correctly by men, it increases sperm count, thus enhancing fertility.

8. GTF Chromium:

As the name implies, this is a compound molecule of the earth element chromium, which is found naturally in our body. This molecule is mostly anti-diabetic in function. Yes, you heard right. GTF Chromium helps make insulin more effective in the body and also cuts down blood sugar.

High blood sugar is a major destroyer of tissues and so contributes in a big way to the acceleration of the aging process. Take this supplement in the recommended dosage to control the dedicated attacks of sugar on body cells. This supplement is particularly important if you regularly consume sugar and other such sweet things because it practically lowers the risks of diabetes and keeps the skin looking younger and fresher, free from the signs of aging.

Note the wonder of nature here: Chromium is the same element that is industrially used to transform ordinary steel to high-grade stainless steel!

Hesperidin:

The peels of citrus fruits (orange, lime, grapes, etc.) have powerful insecticide properties but right in there is to be found a specific bioflavonoid which has some astonishing effects on your body as a supplement.

As we age, our veins become bent out of shape. They begin to look like discolored worm-like sprouting under the skin, and depending on your complexion, these sprouting can take many odd colors from purple to green. This supplement increases the tightness of veins, thereby improving blood flow.

Studies have shown that the inflammation in the veins are also reduced markedly with the intake of Hesperidin, so we say this supplement helps to keep your heart young and healthy.

9. Idebenone:

Fondly called the showbiz drug, this supplement is an antioxidant that is the secret behind the youthful looking skin of many aged celebrities down in Hollywood.

When taken on a daily basis, this powerful antioxidant penetrates very deeply into the skin and repairs the terrible damage caused by aging. This wonder of a supplement is to be found in many anti-aging creams the world over. They come quite expensive, though.

10. Imedeen:

This is another wonder drug that is quickly gaining popularity for showing amazing results. It is a protein gotten solely from a deep-sea fish and its contents are known to enhance, or rather, increase the production of elastin and collagen in the human body. These two substances are vital for keeping the skin tight and firm – youthful looking.

Take this supplement daily to help in the provision of hyaluronic acid, a natural moisturizer that does away with free radicals and keeps your skin lithe, soft, and wrinkle free.

10. Heliocare:

This supplement is a fern extract that is highly efficient in protecting the skin from the terrible effects of the sun's ultraviolet rays and the adverse effects of aging.

Take supplementary pills of this drug to lower UVA related damage to the skin while its anti-wrinkle properties efficiently go to work, reducing and prolonging the appearance of pigmentation and wrinkles on the skin.

16. ESSECSIAL OILS FOR ANTI-AGING

For thousands of years, man has exploited the therapeutic and healing properties of essential oils as part of the practice of aromatherapy. These sweet-smelling oils are mostly gotten from the stems, leaves, or roots of plants that are known for unique health properties.

Unique essential oils like frankincense, myrrh, lavender, and sandalwood are among the most effective anti-aging remedies known to man. Until recently, they very rare and expensive. Frankincense is the most unique of the lot, little wonder it was given as a precious gift by the three wise men to the newborn baby, Jesus Christ

These oils are very rich in antioxidants and certain other compounds that balance the body's hormones levels naturally. Most importantly of all is their ability to reduce damages in body cells.

Frankincense Oil

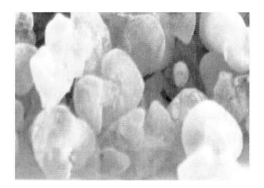

Frankincense (also called Olibanum) is a magical health oil gotten from the resin of the Boswellia sacara tree that's native Somalia, East Africa. This tree is unique in that it can grow in rocky areas with very little soil and under dry and desolate conditions.

Frankincense oil is utilized by either inhaling, absorption through the skin by mixing it in with a carrier agent, such as a lotion or another oil. Some claim frankincense transmits signals to the limbic system of the brain, which influences the nervous system. When ingested, a drop or two of this oil goes a long way. Do not consume any more than this as it can be very toxic.

Frankincense oil is one of the best stress relievers known to man. Just adding two drops to a hot bath and soaking in it will kill off all the pain in the body. It also helps with anxiety, bringing relief to the entire body. Frankincense possesses antiseptic properties that make it the perfect house cleaner. It gets rid of bacteria and viruses in your home, disinfects indoor spaces and deodorizes them all. It also helps oral hygiene, boosts the immune system and digestive system, and fights skin aging with a vengeance! Where ever the wrinkles or sagging, flesh appears, mix six drops of Frankincense oil and one ounce of any unscented oil and apply directly. This oil is so good that its benefits are vast so it's best to use it to maintain overall health – prevention of illnesses is better than cure.

Take just 2 drops of frankincense orally each day. Add it to your drinking water and it boosts your health and slows down the aging process markedly but never forget that this natural anti-aging serum has the best effects when used just before bedtime.

Avocado oil

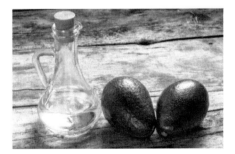

Another important oil here is avocado oil, which has already been dealt with previously. Avocado oil is rich in antioxidants, nutrients, vitamins, minerals and essential fats, all of which make it a very potent anti-aging weapon.

Most of the essential fatty acids contained in avocado oil are monounsaturated oleic acid, very rare omega-9 EFA. Oleic acid works wonders throughout the body – lowering the risk of different kinds of cancers, preventing the development of certain autoimmune diseases, promoting cell regeneration and healing of wounds, boosting the body's resistance and ability to eliminate microbial infections, cutting down inflammation inside and outside the body…these and much more are the work of this unique acid.

Avocado oil, with its high anti-inflammatory properties, boosts the cardiovascular system, overall heart health and lowers blood pressure. Avocado oil also furnishes the body with the ability to convert most of that unhealthy fats in the body into forms of more healthy and usable fats, thanks to its high concentration of beta-sitosterol, which is a type of cholesterol. Throw in that oleic acid and what you got is good news indeed for overweight people looking to slim down and avoid heart diseases.

Avocado oil, like most oils of its kind, is rich in vitamin E which gives it the ability to boost brain, skin, eyes, and heart health. It also boosts the immune system, digestive system, and the body's detox system.

Did I mention that this oil wipes out skin rashes and itching? Yes, the benefits of this oil are endless and it is even better than the avocado fruit itself which has certain unwelcome side effects in the body.

Olive Oil

Firstly, the olive oil being referred to here is not the ordinary kind which is high in harmful fats like most other oils. The variety we are talking of here is the Organic Extra-Virgin Olive Oil. This is the oil that you want.

Original Olive Oil is produced from olives, the fruit of a natural tree that reaches maturity through decades, though that has been remedied by modern science. The natural olive tree is native to the Asia minor and the middle-east region where its unique health and medicinal properties have been well known and well used for more than 4,000 years. The Bible makes too many references to the health and healing properties of this golden oil to be ignored. Right from ancient times, olive oil has been renowned for its ability to heal, preserve and even enhance beauty and youthfulness.

Today, some of the best quality olive oil come from Greece and California, USA, where the trees are grown. Scientists have also found out why this oil has been so famous since ancient time.

Olive oil is super rich in Omega-9 fatty acids which is also known oleic acid (this gives it a lot of unique healing and anti-aging properties similar to avocado oil), vitamin E (olive oil is the best-known source of this very important vitamin) and other important nutrients that make it wonderful on the skin and body organs. Extra virgin Olive Oil is also a wonderful source of certain monounsaturated fats, which helps the cardiovascular system, eyes, skin, and heart.

Are you someone that loves fried foods? Now your seen reason to replace your normal vegetable oil or frying oil with olive oil today! Why?

Go get the olive oil. Not only will the foods taste much better, your health will get much better too.

17. HONEY

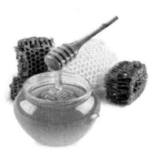

The amazing health benefits of honey are without end. Since good health is good life and longevity, there is a lot that could be talked about here but let's keep things restricted to the subject of anti-aging so as not to create an encyclopedia-sized report out of one single chapter – honey is simply that good!

The Complete Composition of Honey

Honey, the excretion of bees, is made up of sugar (about 76%), water (18%) and other lesser ingredients that account for just about 6% of its composition. Sugar gives the honey its characteristic sweetness while water liquefies all the other components in the substance. These components, though so small in their amounts, are so important that they not only determine the differences between various types of honey – the color, taste, and aroma – but also gives honey its immense health and anti-aging benefits.

1. Sugars

There are actually three different kinds of sugar present in honey - fruit sugar (fructose) 41%, grape sugar (glucose) 34%, ordinary sugar (sucrose) 2%. These ratios of components differ in honey, depending on the source (i.e. is it from flowers or other places), the bees and the existing amounts of the enzyme, invertase, which breaks down regular sugar in grape and fruit. This enzyme invertase, though found in the flowers from which bees collect nectar to form the honey, is also present in the body of the bees themselves.

2. Water

This second highest constituent of honey is there to keep the other ingredients in a soluble state. Water is good for our health, no doubt, but in this case, it acts more like an agent in the way it facilitates the availability of the other ingredients of honey in liquid form for the easy absorption of the body.

3. Other Ingredients of Honey

The other smaller but extremely important ingredients of honey are as follows: proteins, minerals, acids, and unknown matter. The components differ in ratio from one kind of honey to the other.

Minerals

Minerals make up just about 3.69% of honey. Although this part of honey may seem insignificant, it is more than enough to make a huge impact on human health. Honey contains potassium, calcium, copper, chlorine, sodium, sulfur, magnesium, iron, silicon, manganese, and phosphorus, all of which are so important to the body's perfect health. Honey of the dark kind are generally richer in minerals than lighter ones but there are those rare occasions when this does not hold true.

Proteins

The proteins in honey get in there from nectar and pollen which are vital parts of plants. These proteins may be very complex in structure or just simple compounds – amino acids are a good example.

Acids

Until recently, it was thought that bees injected their venom into the cells in the honeycomb where the honey is stored in other to conserve it. Given that formic acid is the main components of bee venom, it was assumed that honey contained the same acid and so was avoided by many people. Studies have since proven that completely different acids are contained in honey, the same acids are found in apples and lemon acid.

Vitamins

Honey has a very modest quantity of vitamins which are actually insufficient for the general needs of the body. Vitamin C, vitamin E and some B complex vitamins (riboflavin, pantothenic acid, biotin, pyridoxine, nicotinic acid).

Essential oils

Both the aroma and somewhat sticky nature of honey are as a result of some essential oils present in it. However, due to the unstable nature of these oils, they quickly evaporate when honey is heated in any manner.

Honey and The Anti-Aging War

No one can tell you that much about the other small part of honey that contains substances that are as yet uncategorized, but that honey has a big impact on health and longevity is no news now. Take two spoonsful of honey daily to start reaping these immense health benefits. When you start adding honey to your drinking water on a daily basis, you get a syrup that works wonders in you.

Honey Is Not Ordinary Sugar

Honey is full of sugar, so why should I dump it in my water daily? How can honey be healthy when it's so sugary?

People ask these and many other questions when they first come to know about the health benefits of honey.

Do not be fooled. Honey is actually so good for you, it is very expensive in most third world countries where this fact is well known. Drinking a glass of warm honey water every day will generally increase your health levels with the short-term effect of making your body more flexible and energetic during exercise routines (the athlete's secret). This will add days to your life and even protect you against many chronic diseases.

The Health Magic of Honey

Like with most sugary fruits, honey does not harm you when eaten daily. The following are what will happen if you start taking honey or adding honey to your drinking water, on a daily basis…

1. Your Gas Will Be Reduced

So many people suffer from bloated tummy, and so gassing is a major problem. If you fall into this category, then a glass of warm honey water will neutralize the gas in your system right where you stand. In no time, you'll feel the relief and lightness within you.

2. Immune System Booster

This is one sweet sugar that can impressively boost your immune system and clear out all those harmful organisms like bacteria and fungus, that affect it. Take honey raw and in its organic form to reap maximum benefit from its bacteria, fungus, and virus killing properties! Honey is loaded with enzymes, minerals, and vitamins that will protect you against the nastiest of bacteria (though some virus may get past it).

3. Toxins Are Flushed Out of Your Body

You can't do much better than honey and warm water for rapid flushing out of toxins (poisons) from your system. Water and honey are a team that tops the list of body detox agents. Your days of troubles with toxins are now over. Say hello to detox and a clean system – adding lemon or lime will give you even better results. Don't be scared if your body starts pumping out urine so much after drinking this mixture, you won't believe how much bad stuff there is to be cleared out of your system! Just keep the urine flowing and never fear! Oh, and don't forget to drink lots and lots of water to promote the detox process and replace all the ones going out of you so fast.

4. Your Skin Becomes Clearer

Honey, having powerful antioxidant and antibacterial properties like it does, will not tolerate free radicals, toxins, wastes or any such harmful substance in your body. It will attack them and flush them all out, thereby keeping both your system and skin clearer than ever. Ever heard of a DIY honey exfoliator? Just take the honey and warm water and forget the big words!

5. Weight Loss

The sugar in honey is totally different from processed white sugar – it is natural sugar! These natural sugars in honey will not only satisfy your daily craving for sugary treats such as chocolate, cake, sweets, and cola but will also lower that addiction to sugar drastically. Why not substitute your sugar packed drinks with honey water and save yourself the addition of up to 65% more calories to your weight!

6. Fixes Your Sore Throat

In many cold lands, warm honey water is a winter favorite not just because it keeps you warm in the cold months but because it can also soothe sore throat and other illnesses like coughs. Honey is a natural remedy for almost all respiratory infections, so next time you have a cold, reach out for raw honey and not the doctor.

7. Regulates Blood Sugar Levels

As pointed out earlier, while honey contains a good amount of sugar, it's not the same as processed white sugar which has been bleached to give it that attractive white color (sugar comes naturally as a dirty brown substance not white). Honey's unique combination of natural sugars in the form of fructose and glucose are unique in the way they help the body regulate its blood sugar levels. Cholesterol levels are even lowered as well. This is good news indeed for diabetic patients.

8. Lowers Risk of Heart Disease and Other Related Illnesses

Honey contains powerful antioxidants and flavonoids that reduce and even prevent the risk of heart disease. It is now a proven medical fact that honey slows down the oxidation process of bad cholesterol in human blood – the very reaction which leads to heart attacks and strokes.

The Anti-Aging Atom Bomb

Vegetables and fresh fruits topped off with good quality lean beef cuts will make you a wall balanced diet that has very positive effects on your health but add honey in the water you drink to go with this food and its nutrimental value rockets off the charts. These are first-class minerals, vitamins, and hydration packed into your body in one go, and hey, it's an anti-aging atom bomb!

18. ALOE VERA

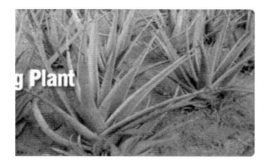

Aloe Vera, the most powerful and versatile anti-aging plant on earth, is known to many as a 'miracle plant' or 'natural healer'. In holding with nature's uncanny ways which place some of the most amazing health remedies in the most unusual places such as animal and incest excreta (e.g. honey from bees), weeds and the parts of foods humans normally throw away such as the barks and peels (e.g. resveratrol in skin of grapes), Aloe Vera is actually a weed. A short and very unattractive weed at that!

Aloe Vera (Aloe Barbadensis Miller), due to its immense health benefits to mankind, is the most important member of the Aloe family which has over 400 species. Aloe Vera means 'True Aloe' and this wonderful plant is actually native to the dry desert lands of North Africa, but its unique ability to survive in any climate and condition, coupled with its renowned health properties, has seen it transplanted all over the world through many centuries.

Indeed, mankind has exploited Aloe Vera for over 3,000 years and wars have even been fought over it!

Descriptions of this miracle plant have been found in the writings of physicians from different cultures and civilizations dating as far back as the ancient Greek, Egyptian, and Roman eras. Ancient Chinese and Indian cultures also describe the powers of Aloe Vera in writings. The earliest record of Aloe Vera is to be found on an ancient stone tablet of Sumerian origin which dates back to 2100 BC! This clearly indicates that the immense therapeutic and healing benefits of Aloe Vera have been well-known since prehistoric times, firmly putting the use of this plant as far back as 4000 years ago!

The Bible makes reference to Aloe Vera, and legend is not left out. Alexander the Great, conqueror of the world all of 2000 years ago, attacked and took the island of Socotra in the Indian Ocean in order to provide his physicians with unlimited access to large supplies of Aloe Vera plants to treat battle wounded soldiers. At the time, Aloe Vera, a crop imported nearly a hundred years before, was growing so abundantly on the Socotra isles, it was regarded as a problematic weed!

The first documented discovery of Aloe Vera's incredible antiquity was actually made in 1862 after an Egyptian papyrus (ancient paper-like document) dated 1550 BC came to light. This document associated the use of Aloe Vera to the physical beauty of Egyptian Queens.

With the ancients clamoring so much about this ugly plant, let's take a closer look at what the noise is all about.

The Unique Health Powers of Aloe Vera

Yes, this plant is an unattractive weed, but this particular weed has the power to heal the body in ways that can only be described as magical.

Indeed, Aloe Vera's unique health and healing powers have made it one of the most popular houseplants in certain parts of the world today and when people get hurt, like with burns or minor wounds, they go grabbing a piece of the plant, extract its gel and massage it into the affected area. That's it! In little time, without pain, Aloe Vera will make that wound disappear without leaving a trace!

Although modern medicine does not give proper recognition to Aloe Vera's unique qualities, traditional medicine and profit-minded cosmetic companies do. In the

Philippines, Aloe Vera is effectively used along with milk to cure kidney infections while over in Japan it is widely used as an ingredient in commercially produced yogurt and beverages. A visit to any cosmetic store in the world will reveal a whole range of Aloe Vera based beauty, skin care, and hair maintenance products.

In this chapter, we will not only learn about the unique benefits of Aloe Vera to human health but also how to reap those benefits all by ourselves and look younger.

The Structure of The Aloe Vera Plant

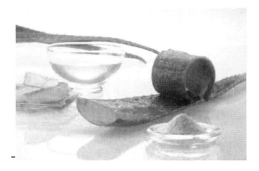

An understanding of the unique structure of this plant is important in the acquisition of knowledge of its use.

Aloe Vera is a very delicate green plant with a short stem. It can grow to between 60 – 100 cm high but its spear-like leaves can reach up to 50 cm or more in length. The leaves are swollen thick and when broken, a sticky colorless gel is found stuffed within.

The Rind is the protective green outer layer of the plant and just within it is the sap, a thin layer of extremely bitter fluid that makes the plant very unpleasant as food to animals, hence they will never eat it. That colorless gel stuffed in the inner part of the thick leaf is called Mucilage Gel and it is the part that is filleted out (or gouged out – depending on how you do it) to become the all-super healing gel.

Aloe Vera gel is the most vital part of the plant health-wise. In addition to its impressive antibacterial, antiviral and antifungal properties, this gel contains the 18 important Amino Acids needed by the human body, 8 of which are hardly ever there because the body cannot manufacture them by itself. Other constituents of Aloe Vera include the B complex vitamins and Vitamin C, thrown in with the other important acids, they make this ordinary looking Aloo Vera gel a potent anti-aging tool that attacks free radicals throughout the body.

Ingested externally through the skin, Aloe Vera works its wonders. But it also works more wonders when consumed orally, so if you can't overcome the terrible bitter taste, some fruit juice and honey might help make it more palatable.

Aloe Vera gel is not to be confused with Aloe Vera juice. The juice, which is of far lesser health benefit to mankind, is gotten from the sap while the super healing gel is what is naturally packed into the leaf to make it so thick.

12 Essential Uses and Remedies of Aloe Vera

The first thing to note here is that Aloe Vera does not store well and so is best used when extracted freshly from the plant. An alternative is to buy the natural gel or juice as a preserved product, they come mostly in tubes, but you need to be careful there because the gel and juice in those tubes are packed with chemicals to preserve it.

So now you know more about Aloe Vera, below are some benefits of its use and how to exploit them directly at home.

1. Healing of minor wounds

For centuries, Aloe Vera gel has been used for external treatment of burns, minor wounds, and skin irritations. Aloe Vera used to be known as the 'burn plant' due to its magical cure of burns. Break open the leave, extract the gel and apply on the affected area of skin and you'll be fine. This plant's gel has the power to heal wounds without leaving scars.

2. Controls and Cures Irritable Bowel Syndrome

Taken orally in its fresh and raw form, Aloe Vera gel has a marked effect on Irritable Bowel Syndrome (IBS) – a dedicated 2-year trial involving 44 patients suffering from Ulcerative Colitis at the Royal London Hospital in Oxford, England; stumbled upon this discovery in 2004.

3. Cures Respiratory Infections

One of the most popular home remedies for asthma and respiratory tract infections is to boil a few Aloe Vera leaves in a bowl of water and breathe in the vapor of the brew.

4. Cures Skin Diseases

Aloe Vera is also remarkable in the treatment of Eczema and Psoriasis.

5. Used as A Laxative

For medicinal use as a laxative, Aloe juice is used. It actually comes from the tubules just beneath the outer skin of the thick leaves and is very different from the gel.

6. Universal Cure for Diseases

Make Aloe Vera into a beverage or add a spoonful of the gel to a cup of green tea, sweetened with honey. Drink this mixture twice a day to cure or control any of the following conditions, constipation, headaches, ulcers, arthritis, diabetes, and coughs.

Warning! With certain people, internal consumption of Aloe Vera could have some side effects such as stomach pain, diarrhea or electrolyte imbalances. None of these issues are fatal and, in most cases, they disappear with continuous consumption of Aloe Vera, but it is best you know how your body could react to your intake of this powerful substance even if for the first time. So, take very little of it the first time to check. This issue will be clarified later after you get a better idea of the dosages of Aloe Vera gel considered safe for consumption.

7. Fights Irritation

Are you a woman suffering from vaginal irritations? Give Aloe Vera a try before rushing off to the doctor. Massage a generous amount of the gel into the affected area twice a day and it will even help get rid of virginal odor.

8. Internal Sore Treatments

Aloe Vera may be used to treat mouth sores, stomach sores of all kinds, and even cold sores. Just consume the gel orally as a beverage and relax. But with mouth sores, if you can stand the bitter taste, massage the gel directly into the affected area.

9. Universal Cure for Skin Diseases

Aloe Vera gel is nature's gift to patients with various kinds of skin diseases. It rejuvenates, moisturizes and hydrates the skin. How? After being rubbed on, Aloe Vera gel penetrates deeply into the skin (several layers deeper than any other cosmetic) and stimulates the fibroblasts cells in a way that causes them to regenerate faster. These cells then produce elastin and collagen which literally injects new life into the skin, causing it to become very fresh, smooth and youthful looking.

10. Bowel Disease Prevention and Gastrointestinal Tract Detox

Aloe Vera not only helps in the cure of irritable bowel syndrome as pointed out above but it cuts down the risks of this disease ever occurring to you. This is possible because, Aloe Vera, with its unique vitamins and minerals, is a natural substance that works gently and systematically within the stomach (bowels) and intestinal tract. It helps break down food residues that have become stuck in the walls of the stomach and intestine, and thus, cleans them out When the stomach (bowel), the larger organ, is thoroughly cleaned out in this manner, it greatly decreases stomach bloating, discomfort, and stress, all of which lead to attacks of irritable bowel syndrome. (See research information on digestive system detox in next section below).

11. Anti-Aging Weapon and Immune System Booster

Aloe Vera is rich in polysaccharides that boost the immune system. Its high antioxidants content guarantee that it is always at war, both inside and outside the body, with all those substances that enhance aging, e.g. free radicals, other harmful chemicals, and toxins.

12. Maintains A Very Beneficial Alkaline system

Oral consumption of Aloe Vera maintains the alkalinity of your system and this neutralizes all the acidic substances and organisms that foster bad health and the aging process. Sugar, for example, is acidic once in the body and so this quality of Aloe Vera can be called an anti-diabetic one. A lot of other harmful organisms and body processes, which flourish in acidic systems, leading to diseases and illness are eliminated.

Aloe Vera: A Miracle Skin Care tool

The greatest attribute of any anti-aging substance is its ability to keep the skin looking much younger and fresher. In this regard, Aloe Vera is a champion! There is no other substance on earth like it.

Aloe Vera fights wrinkles

Aloe Vera gel is well known as a wonderful remedy for sunburns. But that's only the tip of the iceberg!

According to a study conducted by some researchers and published in the prestigious Annals of Dermatology in early 2009, just ¼ teaspoon (1200 mg/dosage) of pure and natural Aloe Vera gel can markedly reverse all signs of skin aging within the period pf **90 days**!

They figured this out by subjecting 30 healthy women, all above the age of 45 years, to the reception of 2 different oral doses of Aloe Vera for 90 days.

*Low dose – 1200 mg/dosage.

*High dose – 3600 mg/dosage

After the period of just 90 days, facial wrinkles significantly faded away in both groups, but, for some reason, the group with a lower dosage had better facial elasticity.

To say this result was astonishing is an understatement. It highlighted the fact that the body does not do well with the internal consumption of high doses of Aloe Vera gel. Anything over a quarter (¼) of a teaspoon a day is over the safe dosage.

The evidence was right there and the discovery unique: The production of collagen in the body increased with daily consumption (drinking) of this safe dosage of Aloe Vera gel – collagen is the basic structural component of the skin and so the more collagen produced by your body, the less wrinkles and sagging flesh you have.

The most amazing discovery of all was that Aloe Vera worked way down at basic DNA levels to cut down all gene activity that caused the destruction of collagen in the first place!

Other discoveries made, gave insight to the powerful detoxing properties of Aloe Vera. This quality of Aloe Vera has actually been known and exploited for ages, but the researchers gave adequate explanations for the process.

Aloe Vera: A Powerful Detoxing agent

Apart from its ability to rejuvenate the skin, Aloe Vera rejuvenates other areas of the body too by its unique detox properties.

Digestive System Detox

Aloe Vera can detox the digestive system with wonderful results. After consumption, the gel is not broken down but moves through the digestive and intestinal tract, picking up toxins all the way. It drags them all out of the body through the colon (anus) and that's the end of the poisons in your body.

Body Detox

Consumed orally, Aloe Vera has the ability to detox your entire body system in a way that makes your skin glow with health and beauty. Working from the inside out, Aloe Vera injects new life into your aged skin, reversing things completely.

The 3 Unique Benefits of Aloe Vera To the Skin

These 3 unique benefits of Aloe Vera on the body's largest organ, as highlighted by this research, definitely makes it the ultimate anti-aging plant.

1. Applied directly on the skin, it repairs all damage (wounds, burns, acne, scars).

2. Ingested internally it helps rebuild collagen (much of it is produced and faster too).

3. Aloe Vera works at basic DNA level in its fights to prevent the destruction of highly essential collagen in the first place.

Put in simple terms, Aloe Vera works from within the body outwards to reverse wrinkles and prevent new ones from forming – you get to look a lot younger within 90 days!

Homemade Aloe Vera Remedies

Aloe Vera is the only safe, nontoxic and natural anti-aging remedy – it also counts as one of the cheapest ever! Indeed, while chemical laden beauty and skin care cosmetic products that give you the desired youthful look are so expensive, Aloe Vera, pure and natural, is free! You just need to know how to use it to get the perfect results and this is where homemade remedies come in.

For homemade remedies, you need the actual Aloe Vera plant around you, at home. Plant it in your garden, or in a vase if you live in an apartment, and it will take care of itself, thanks to its 'all climate survival' abilities as a weed. If you can lay hands on the plant from other sources, then lucky you.

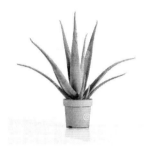

Once you get your hands on the plant, what you do then is extract that miracle gel from inside the thick leaf. This extraction process is easy and once done, you've got one of the cheapest and most powerful anti-aging weapons in your hands!

This sticky colorless gel is very precious indeed. Although 96% water, it contains over 200 healing phytonutrients and then some more healers. In case you have to get the Aloe Vera leaf from somewhere, it possible to store it in the fridge. It will stay fresh for about 14 to 21 days.

Warning!

Ensure you do not use any store-purchased Aloe Vera gel because to preserve it, the manufacturing companies add in lots of chemicals and non-edible nasty stuff.

So, you've now got the miracle working Aloe Gel, time to get going on some fast working remedies all by yourself.

1. Basic Aloe Vera Remedies for Skin Preservation

For a basic fix of most skin problems using Aloe Vera gel remedies, which will also work to preserve the skin, the following is all you need do.

1. Rub a good amount of your freshly harvested organic Aloe gel on a chosen part of your skin. Massage it carefully into the skin in circular motions for about 3 minutes and it will be absorbed completely.

Do this each day to your face before bedtime to help get rid of toxins and tone facial skin even as it is injected full of nourishing and healing ingredients.

Also, apply the gel over and around the eyes – Aloe Vera is actually known to be the most potent eye cream ever.

2. For areas where wrinkles have already taken root, mix 1 teaspoon full of Aloe Vera gel with a capsule of Vitamin E. Apply directly to those areas (if you can't get vitamin E capsules make do with Extra Virgin Olive Oil which is rich in it).

3. To keep the skin looking young, it's important to promote the production of collagen and halt its destruction. Add ¼ teaspoon of Aloe Vera gel to your daily beverage and you'll be better than fine,

2. Aloe Vera For Eye Problems

To combat the problem of puffy eyes and dark circles around the eyes, which are both caused by under-eye wrinkles, pure Aloe Vera gel is there for you. This gel is easily absorbed into the skin, penetrating deeply to soothe the affected areas like nothing else can. It's truly the best way.

In this case, you may choose to use the natural Aloe Vera gel alone or mix it with an equal portion of sweet almond oil. Whichever you choose, apply it very carefully to the delicate under eye skin. Using your fingers, gently tap the mixture or gel into your skin until it's fully absorbed. Try not to rub the gel in vigorously because this can promote more wrinkles on the delicate under-skin.

Do this often before bedtime and the eyes problems will be history.

3. Aloe Vera Scrub for Skin Defoliation

Skin defoliation refers to the important process of removing dead cells from the outer layers of the skin, particularly the face. Regular exfoliation promotes skin cell turnover (energy output) and increases overall collagen production.

Injecting Aloe Vera gel into this exfoliation process works wonders. Try this remedy below.

Ingredients for Remedy
- 1 tablespoonful of natural Aloe Gel
- 1 tablespoonful of natural olive oil (extra virgin)
- ¼ cupful of brown natural sugar

Get and mix up these ingredients together. Massage it carefully and gently into the skin of your face in circular motions. Do this unhurriedly for about 4 to 5 minutes then relax for about 2 minutes more before rinsing off with warm water. You should feel the freshness of your face even as you pat the skin dry with a towel.

The brown natural sugar will exfoliate (remove) all the dead skin, allowing Aloe Vera's healing nutrients and the vitamin E rich olive oil penetrate deeply into your skin.

Do these 3 times a week for best results, which are beautiful skin, and glowing complexion.

4. Aloe Vera Face Mask to Make You Look Younger

Clean off the skin of your face and neck with clean warm water before applying any facial mask. Get rid of all cosmetics, lotions, creams, everything! If it's possible for you to take a hot, pore-opening, steaming shower –better. When done, apply the face mask right off.

Ingredients
*1 teaspoonful of Aloe Vera gel

* A Pinch of Turmeric Powder

* 1 teaspoonful of milk

* 1 teaspoonful of raw honey

* Just a few drops of Rose Water

Mix all these ingredients together without the Aloe Vera gel. Make a paste of them before adding up the Aloe

Vera gel. Now mix the whole thing very well and then apply the mixture evenly over the skin of your neck and face. Leave it on for 15 to 20 minutes and then wash it all off with warm water. Pat your skin dry carefully with a clean towel.

Repeat this process just once each week and within the first month, others will start talking about your 'new youthful looks!

5. Simple Aloe Vera Face Mask

Some of the ingredients used above are difficult to get ahold of so alternatively, you can try a simpler form of this homemade Aloe Vera face mask:

Ingredients

* 1 tablespoon of Aloe Vera gel.

*1 teaspoonful of seaweed powder

Mix them together without adding water and then apply a thin layer to the skin of your face and neck. Leave it on for about 10 to 12 minutes before rinsing off with lukewarm water. Try to do this at least once a week.

Note – in addition to the stimulation of blood circulation, Seaweed powder helps markedly to detoxify the body, getting rid of impurities and nourishing the skin by injecting it with vital nutrients. This process leaves your skin glowing richly with health.

5b. Another Alternative Aloe Face Mask (the best)

Here is yet another alternative to the two face masks above. Funnily, it actually gives a result far better than both.

Ingredients

* 1 teaspoonful of Aloe Vera gel

* 1 teaspoonful of olive oil.

* 1 egg yolk

Make a mixture of these thick ingredients and apply it carefully on your face. Leave for about 20 minutes and then rinse off with warm water. This face mask is simply awesome in performance. It will have you looking like you've taken a Botox injection to look way younger. I kid you not!

5c. Alternative Face Mask

This is another alternative Aloe face mask remedy.

Ingredients

*1/2 cup of fresh grapes juice

* 1 tablespoon of Aloe Vera gel

* 1 tablespoon of raw honey.

Put it all in a blender to make a paste. Apply the mixture evenly over your face and neck, leave for 20 minutes, rinse off with lukewarm water and pat dry with a clean towel. Do this once a week.

Pick your choice of the face masks with respect to the ingredients within reach, make it and start looking younger already. Once you coat your skin with the mixture, take your time and relax, watch some TV or read a magazine. Whatever you do, just be sure to give the mask time to work on your skin before you rinse off. You may even choose to place 2 slices of cucumber on your eyes – alternatively, use 2 used and cooled chamomile tea bags, or 2 cotton pads which have been soaked in lavender or rose water. This will soothe the eyes deeply and have it looking clearer, this translates into better eyesight.

6. Aloe Vera Facial Spray

First of all, get rid of that toxic industrially manufactured face spray you are already using, then relax and enjoy the soothing and hydrating benefits of Aloe Vera and rosewater – anywhere, anytime.

Ingredients for Remedy

*1 teaspoonful of Aloe Vera gel

* 1 fresh cucumber

* 2 teaspoonfuls of rosewater

* 1 bottle of natural mineral water

*Get a neat spray bottle.

Peel off the green bark of the cucumber and put it in a blender to make a paste. Use a fine sieve, or just strain, to get all the juice from that paste into a bowl. Add all the other ingredients mentioned above, except the mineral water, to the juice and mix well. Now, carefully transfer this "mixed juice" into the clean spray bottle and add that mineral water.

Congratulations! Your pleasant-smelling spray is now ready for use. Your very own nontoxic Aloe Vera facial spray! Spray it on a few times a day. Although this spray can be stored in a fridge for up to a week or two, due to its wonderful nature, you might finish it long before then.

Final Word on Aloe Vera

Aloe Vera works both from the outside in and the inside out to keep you looking, not just younger and healthier, but fresher!

Now that you've come to understand the unique powers of Aloe Vera, which had all those ancient people from Greece, Egypt and Rome screaming, there's still need for caution before you go rushing out the door to get the biggest tube of Aloe Vera gel or the largest Aloe Vera plant that catches your eye:

1. Species Blunder

There are over 400 species of Aloe in the world, and species tend to look very much alike. That huge Aloe Vera plant just down the road could just be something else entirely.

Aloe Barbadensis Miller is the plant you want. Aloe Vera meaning 'True Aloe', is the most popular specie of the entire Aloe family but can be easily mistaken for another. Try not to make such mistake. Locate the real plant and get it planted in your garden at home for ready use. Alternatively, you can just buy a 100% pure organic Aloe Vera gel or juice.

2. Pay Careful Attention to Dosage

As pointed out before, Aloe Vera gel is one natural substance that doesn't bear the right results with the oral consumption of high dosages. High amounts of Aloe in the body can cause allergic reactions or even diarrhea. The safest dosage of Aloe Vera the body needs on a daily basis is ¼ of a teaspoon. This is enough to give you all the amazing anti-aging benefits we've talked about here so avoid the temptation of increasing dosage to avoid toxicity.

3. Certain people are allergic to Aloe Vera gel.

True, some individuals are sensitive or even allergic to Aloe Vera and so cannot really use it on their skin or take it orally. If you are using Aloe Vera for the first time, do this – rub a small amount of the gel on a small part of your skin and look out for negative reactions.

Aloe Vera, the miracle plant, turns back the clock on your aged skin by promoting the production of new collagen and preventing the breakdown of existing ones. No other plant in nature can do this and no medical process can.

Give Aloe Vera a try today and in little time, people will be asking about the gifted plastic surgeon doing you up to look so good!

19. WATER

Our body is made up mostly of water and so we need to consume a lot it daily to replenish all that which has been lost through urination, sweating, and other means. Water is good for you, that's a fact. Drinking plenty of water will help you stay hydrated, help your kidneys and liver flush out toxins from your body and improve your digestive system. Your skin, which is also a means for removing toxins from your body through sweating, will be deep cleaned and kept healthy.

Water is indeed a vital component in our body. All the minerals and nutrients we consume, all the supplements, they would all be useless without water! Why? Water, a universal solvent, essentially maintains all the body's daily functions, from the transportation of important nutrients, minerals, and oxygen to facilitating digestion of food.

There is no end to our body's need for water and so we should be drinking more and more of it each day! It may not have direct anti-aging properties but without water the anti-aging foods we eat, the body detox processes, they will not work at all. Lack of water will even make your skin look dry and wrinkled – that's dehydration in effect.

Avoid drinking very cold water as it alters the body's natural temperature balance in a way that not even a cold environment will. You see, even in very cold environments, the body tries to maintain a core temperature in order to keep your organs and system working normally. But drinking very cold water, taking it directly into your body, alters that core temperature. This is the exact opposite of a fever which gets your core temperate hotter than normal. Either way, nothing good comes out of it. It is far better to drink warm water than anything else and below are some reasons why…

Reasons Why You Should Consume Warm Water:

The following are reasons why you should opt for a glass of warm water rather than a glass of chilled water at all times.

1. Body Detoxification

Drink a glass of warm water on an empty stomach each morning to trigger your body's natural detoxification process. This will eliminate all the harmful toxins stored up in your body as a direct result of an unhealthy lifestyle.

2. Promotes Digestion

Water promotes the breakdown of food in the stomach and improves the overall function of the digestive system. It's not cold water, though, but a nice glass of warm water. It will work wonders in your digestive system just that way.

3. Boosts Metabolism

Drink a glass of warm water each morning to boost your metabolism and enhance your body's overall function. Stomachaches, caused by slow metabolic function and improper food digestion, are eliminated swiftly by drinking just a glass of warm water.

4. Eases pain

When in pain, a lot of people get relief by drinking a mere glass of warm water, especially in the case of abdominal pains or menstrual cramps. The extra heat from the water relaxes your stomach muscles, and thus, ease the pain. Other kinds of pain get taken away too because that extra heat improves capillary circulation and relaxes a lot of other tense muscles.

5. Boosts weight loss

Warm water is an excellent weight loss remedy when combined with a healthy diet and regular exercise. That extra heat in warm water increases your body's core temperature just nicely and this speeds up your metabolism, helping your body burn off those problematic calories faster. Your kidneys and all the other excretory organs benefit too.

6. Improves circulation

As already mentioned, drinking warm water on an empty stomach triggers the flushing out of toxins and accumulated waste from your body. This leads to a speed-up of blood circulation (blood flow within the body) and better overall health.

7. Slows down the aging process

Who doesn't want to look beautiful and stay young forever? People will do anything to preserve youth and slow down the aging process. Common water can certainly help achieve this difficult goal by directly preventing premature aging. Toxins and free radicals are the main culprits when it comes to looking much older than your actual age. Drink a glass of warm water first thing every morning, empty as your stomach is, and it will trigger the body's natural ability to eliminate these toxins and free radicals faster. This will ultimately slow down the aging process and improve your overall body health.

20. UNIQUE EXERCISES AND HABITS THAT PROMOTE ANIT-AGING

There's no doubt about it; working out regularly keeps your body younger, both in terms of the energy and physical fitness. Fitness is a youth serum that completely affects how youthful you look, the way you move and the way you feel, your ability physically to do whatever you want, always.

Working out is an anti-aging champion that keeps your body and muscles well-toned and fit. It checks the process of aging which weakens the muscles and skin, making them loose elasticity (become slack), so we need to tighten thing up in other to look good, stay young and feel it too.

Below are some exercising tips to help you stay healthy, agile and youthful looking all through life.

1. Walking and Jogging

Get going right now. Interestingly, there's no need for you to run a hundred miles every day, just start out walking and keep at it for up to 10 minutes a day, then 15, push yourself to 20 minutes, and in no time, you're walking 30 –

45 minutes every day, then one day you break out in a slow run without even realizing it and the jogging begins. If you do not want to jog, then brisk walking will do just fine. Begin slow but **always end fast** so as to eliminate pains from muscle strains due to all that new stress on previously inactive muscles.

Do not forget to do some weight lifting exercises as well. Lift weights 2 – 3 times each week, and what you've got is a simple and easy plan for your body to beat the effects of aging. So many people swear that regular exercise boosts self-confidence and positive mental outlook. They claim to walk taller (more confidently), have better mental clarity (focus), and a general feeling of well-being (feeling so good inside out).

Don't have the energy to start moving your body rapidly through daily exercise routines? Try some honey tonic before you get going. Professional athletes figured out this secret long ago and use it successfully for training routines till date. Take a look above and check out the section for Honey again.

2 Bending Exercise and The Joints

The number one problem with aging is that of painful joints. There is nothing so terrible as having pains in your waist and knees, which stiffen and crack all the time, particularly when you bend over, stand or sit. A lot of my older patients come in and say, 'Please, Doc, I can't bend over, it hurts my waist and knees". I throw my pen carelessly on the floor to one side and tell them to go pick it up, and sure enough, they walk right over, bend right over and pick it up from the floor! What's the point here? You can bend, squat or do anything you want without those pains and stiff joints if you trained you aging body to keep doing things like that. Take Muslims for example, they pray several times a day, standing, kneeling and bending, over and over again on a mat. Go to a big mosque anywhere and take a good look, they are there, thousands of them — older people, some with gray hairs – standing, kneeling and bending over effortlessly alongside very young people! How is this possible? Unknowingly, they have been training their body to do that particular bit of exercise, day in day out, for years!

3. Hack your genetics with resistance training

The saying goes that you cannot change your genes. That's not quite true, though. We can't change our genetic makeup, yes, but we can certainly change how some genes are expressed: how much they do and exactly what they do. One way we do this all the time is strength training. Research has shown that just 30 weeks of resistance training, reverses the aging process at the genetic level. While physical training preserves muscle masses that are typically lost as we get older, it is actually possible to train the body to behave the way it did when it was younger.

4. Do brain workouts too

Your brain, like your body, actually needs exercise too. The more brain-related activity you can do, the better. Try reaction training (such as playing tennis or even the simple throwing and catching of balls), Memorizing choreography or rapid changing of direction like in American dance stepping, kickboxing, and other such recreational activities will do just fine.

5. Make your two brains talk together

Frequently do those exercises where you cross your arms and legs over the midline of your body. Why is that? With aging comes deterioration in the connection between the left and right hemispheres of your brain. This causes "brain delays" as the hemispheres have problems communicating with each another, Fitness experts claim that crossing your limbs forces the two sides of your brain to talk to one another. Well, if so then this bit of workout actually strengthens and preserves the brain, making your overall brain function better.

6. Do more high-impact activity

Older people typically avoid exercises such as running and jumping because they feel it will hurt their feet, knees or hips. Fitness experts claim the contrary is the case. You need to run or jump every day as this high impact activity builds bone density. Don't make a crazy move here, such as breaking into all out runs or doing high jumps. Do thing gently and well within your limit, at least in the beginning. Try some slow and easy military matching moves, or even better, kick a football around in a field and keep going after it.

7. Count your steps as you walk

This is more of a trick to train both the brain and body at the same time. Tracking your steps by giving each a number so fast while you watch where you are headed will have you making mistakes all over the place, and so your brain will upgrade its work rate to cope.

On the average, Americans walk only 2,000 steps per day, but research shows that at least 7,500 steps is required daily for good health. We definitely need to take walking a bit more seriously, particularly stair climbing.

Merely tracking your steps is double exercise., Go get new walking shoes and hit the park. See if you can better the number of steps you take each day and you are on your way to good health and longevity.

8. Sit up straight

Some bad sitting postures actually cause back pains but that is not why this topic is here. Since people with good body postures are often seen as younger, healthier and more confident, sitting up fits in as an anti-aging exercise. Proper sit-up postures eliminate the possibility of joint and muscle pains and can help bypass brain tension and headaches by cutting back strain on the neck.

Yoga routines will help push up your posture by strengthening the muscles in your abdomen, lower back, and pelvis – these muscles are the very ones that help hold your body upright. But it's not only yoga that pays, simply stretching your body very well several times a day will do fine, particularly after long periods of sitting down in one position.

9. Have more sex

Middle-aged people can look up to 10 years younger by just having regular sex.

Researchers in Scotland, going by a 10-year study, found that people in their 40s who enjoy intercourse daily looked at least 12 years younger than those who did this less frequently. The faces and skin of sexually active couples had less stress lines and wrinkles, while the general look of their skin was smoother and suppler. The conclusion was drawn that oxytocin, a stress-reducing chemical released during sex, was responsible for turning back the clock.

Nighttime sex, which helps you sleep deeply so you look and feel very well rested next day, is advised.

Your love life is actually your long life so get busy with your partner at least three times a week. Just tell him or her that it's for their own good health!

21. BIZARE BUT AMAZING ANTI-AGING REMEDIES

The following are some of the strangest remedies taking the health and beauty world by storm today, all with marked anti-aging properties.

Bee venom

A lot of celebrities down in Hollywood swear by this new skin enhancing therapy that claims to revitalize the skin completely.

Breast milk facial

Ever since researchers proved that lauric acid, which is found richly in breast milk, possesses massive anti-inflammatory and antibacterial properties, beauty salons across the USA have gone into a new kind of business called the breast milk facial.

Beer baths

This remedy is much like steam baths. A beer-like mixture of specially-brewed malt, hops, beer yeast, and minerals, is heated to more than 30°C in the presence of the human skin. This deep cleans the skin, sweating away harmful toxins and leaving the skin glowing and reinvigorated

Banana peel

Ever since one Los Angeles beauty blogger revealed how an old banana peel can rejuvenate the skin, there's been much talk about it in the world of beauty and skin care. Apparently, banana peels contain the antioxidant, lutein, a carotenoid closely related to vitamin A. This substance helps diminish inflammation on the skin.'

Urine

And now comes the main event!

Bloggers swear that this disgusting substance, when consumed orally and regularly, has the ability to knock decades off your life, increase longevity and shut down any sickness or disease present in the body. Wow! Amazing news! But before I go drinking gallons of a substance modern medical experts call 'poisonous', is there any proof to the contrary?

First off, it will amaze you to learn that 99.9% of these people calling themselves modern medical experts don't know squat about a lot of things! Take the mind or brain, for example, they still don't know exactly how it works after so many decades and tons of research! They don't even know the exact constituents of honey, and hence, classify about 1% of it as unknown matter. They say the sun's rays are harmful to humans but forget that the body can only get vitamin D by the action of that very harmful sun on the skin. In the case of the immense health benefits of urine, these medical experts have refused to listen at all because the consumption of urine is considered disgusting by themselves and so many other people.

Today, by the standards of western medicine, there is no evidence whatever to support the massive health benefits of urine therapy. But the truth refuses to go away and so certain physicians, like myself, have started paying more attention to urine therapy. We are late, though, because over in Asia, urine therapy is already well established on different levels.

In India, cow urine therapy is already famous for its amazing health benefits. Most Indian villagers live very healthy and disease-free lives by drinking several cups of cow urine daily!

Just recently, a major British media outlet (the BBC) ran the astonishing story of a 36-year-old Indian man, Cement Paliwal, who claimed he and his four friends have been drinking and bathing cow urine for over five years, and it has kept them completely disease free since! The youthful looking men do day jobs at a cow shed in a village in Udaipur, Rajasthan, western India. Cement claims to have turned to cow urine therapy (a very popular remedy in that region) after modern medicine failed to cure him of acute lung diseases that had him catching coughs and colds too regularly.

Cynics may put down all this love for cow urine in this region of Asia to the simple fact that the cow is considered to be the holiest animal on earth by the Hindus and so its milk, and even urine, is considered to have great divine importance. However, this is not the case.

In India, cow urine is known to be a vital ingredient of most medicines – eye and ear drops, joint pain ointments and other such ointments, even antiseptic liquids. The trend of drinking cow urine in its raw form is so popular that major brands are already cashing in on it by selling packed cow urine at prices several times more expensive than vegetable oil!

Interestingly, the overall health benefits of cow urine pales when compared to that of human urine and this brings us to our main subject – the amazing health and anti-aging benefits of human urine.

22. URINE: YOUR BODY'S OWN PERFECT NATURAL MEDICINE

If you think you've heard it all when it comes to fighting diseases by means of natural therapy, you are in for a rude shock this time. Of all the bizarre methods of treatment and therapies you've ever heard of, this one will knock the senses out of you, and get this, it's incredibly old!

This natural therapeutic method is not just the most powerful, but about the most researched, and certainly the most medically proven natural remedies (cures) ever to be discovered.

Irrespective of how hard it may be to believe; the fact remains that knowing the complete truth about this astonishingly powerful natural substance will be the most important health knowledge you'll ever learn. Tighten up your seat belts now as we take an interesting drive down a road that is thousands of years old.

Introduction, History& Definition of Human Urine Therapy

Drink waters out of thine own cistern and running waters out of thine own well.
Proverbs 5:15 (ASV)

Perhaps, this bit of wisdom from the lips of famously wise King Solomon of ancient Israel is the oldest proof there is that urine therapy has been in use since the beginning of human civilization. From this bit of biblical wisdom alone, it is quite clear that urine therapy (the anti-aging secret weapon as some have called it) has proven its potency as a universal cure for illnesses and diseases all of four thousand years ago, making it one of the oldest therapies in the world!

A technique carried down from generation to generation, **Human Urine Therapy** is a drugless, time-proven system of inducing healing and cures for all manner of diseases and sicknesses. Through every civilization from prehistorical times, people have always been aware of the unique 'universal healing' properties of Urine. Aside from this ancient biblical reference to urine, the 'Yogic and Tantric books' (ancient historical and religious records of

Asia, which date as far back as the 5th century), hold several more. That urine therapy is a very old method of treating illnesses is something that is very hard to disprove.

The drinking of urine to treat illnesses and diseases in any form is considered a very unorthodox practice by so many, and this is putting it nicely. Millions of people see it as downright disgusting, but, interestingly, will lick their fingers dry when dipped in honey, which is technically the 'urine' of bees! Although not recognized in the Western world today, human urine therapy is well accepted in the orient.

In China, urine therapy has been in use for hundreds of years, and today, there are hundreds of thousands of people practicing urine therapy on mainland China alone! The China Urine Therapy Association has over 100,000 registered members on the Chinese mainland alone and more elsewhere in Asia. The chairman of the association, 79-year-old *'young guy'* named Bao Yafu, has a daily routine where he drinks three cups of his own urine daily, drops it in his eyes and washes his face with it too! Bao Yafu claims he has not had even a cold in 22 years of doing this, his eyesight is sharp and you'll need a magnifying glass to find the wrinkles anywhere on his face, if any, on his skin. Oh, did I mention he's quite fit and trim? This is the reason I referred to him as a 'young guy'.

For nearly four hundred years, human urine has been very effectively used for both diagnostic and therapeutic purposes in various traditional systems in different parts of the world, but it wasn't until the beginning of the 20th century that the first western doctor took the boldest step of going public with it in western lands. British naturopath John W. Armstrong is to be credited for the initial introduction of urine therapy as a system of alternative medicine in the early 20th century. He was quite successful in his days, with thankful patients in the thousands, but with his death came the end of all formal recognition for urine therapy. Although the use of urine for diagnostic purposes is still well accepted medically today, the therapeutic use of urine is all but dead. This is very baffling indeed considering that there are over 8,000 diseases currently known to man and medical science offers a cure for less than half of that while urine does a lot better.

Indeed, millions of people suffer from countless forms of Chronic Diseases today, most of which are incurable. Mankind is feeling utterly helpless and dejected like never before.

While the number of people afflicted with these terrible diseases is growing each year, scientists and Medical Researchers, despite their tireless endeavors and the cutting-edge medical technology available to them, have failed to discover permanent cures for too many of these illnesses and diseases.

The Wonderful Healing Power Within You

Water, air, and sunlight are all free provisions of nature, which are indispensable to our body. Unknown to many, nature also provides us with a "DIVINE SYRUP" known as "URINE" which flows freely from our bodies. Urine possesses a unique Healing Power that enables it to **Control** and **Cure** all kinds of **Sicknesses** and **Diseases**. In that way, nature has provided very special milk in the breast of a nursing mother for the nourishment of her infant child, so also has nature provided matured human beings with **Urine** for the preservation of health and the cure of all manner of diseases and ailments.

23. URINE THERAPY: MEDICAL RESEARCH AND STANDPOINT

Human urine is merely a purified derivative of the blood produced by the kidneys, which contains, not body waste matter as science says, but an amazing array of extremely important nutrients, hormones, enzymes, natural antibodies and other immune defense agents. – **Dr. Laura Zeaman**

With all the talk about the amazing healing qualities of urine therapy, how incredibly effective and cheap it is, one wonders why the medical community is not promoting it vigorous to the public, particularly given the magnitude of illnesses and diseases afflicting mankind today. In fact, modern doctors and researchers refuse to promote urine therapy in any official manner. This standpoint of the medical community has led to a complete ignorance by the public on the subject of urine therapy. We will now take a close look at this.

Is the Medical Community Aware of The Amazing Healing Qualities of Human Urine?

The answer here is, yes, yes, we are. And we have been in the know for decades!

Medical doctors and scientists, through clinical research and observation, know all about the incredible healing qualities of human urine and they have more details on the subject than most traditional doctors in the Orient who have had the knowledge passed on down to them from generation to generation, for a thousand years. Why do you think medical doctors and workers always ask for the urine of sick patients when carrying out advanced medical tests in search of illness and diseases?

The simple truth of the matter is that human urine is the most amazing proven natural cure ever discovered by medical science. Even the most prestigious doctors and researchers have been stunned by the amazing medical cures witnessed in the clinical use of this incredibly effective and inexpensive substance that is human urine.

This drugless and painless system of healing the body as a whole (urine therapy) is effective against all known diseases and illnesses, except those caused by structural disorders or traumatism. There is really no drug that can equal the power of human urine. What's more? Some of the most expensive drugs you buy in drugstores today are actually made from human urine – it's a billion-dollar industry!

All this knowledge and yet none of it has ever been revealed to the public in any capacity. Simply put, the medical community, of which I am one, has pulled off the biggest hoodwink in the history of mankind.

Why Modern Doctors & Researchers Suppress This Incredible Knowledge

The most extraordinary fact about this unrivaled natural therapy is that the entire medical community of the Western world has been aware of its amazing usefulness for decades, and yet has carefully kept this truth from the general public. Why?

The answer is really simple, we, doctors, value our jobs. Just imagine how empty the hospitals and consulting rooms will be if people learned of what Urine therapy can really do. Secondly, teaching people to drink their own urine in the civilized world we live in today is so primitive sounding that no smart doctor wants to be associated with it. Lastly, while there are numerous pharmaceutical companies ready to give doctors huge financial kickback for prescribing their drugs to patients, such bonuses are not available for prescribing urine therapy.

Simply put, there are no monetary rewards or peace of mind for teaching people what scientists clearly know about urine therapy being the most extraordinary natural healing substance in the world. For this reason, the medical community has chosen to keep this invaluable knowledge a secret. Doesn't matter if that secret is the only health tool on earth that is always available to every human being and never out of reach – financially or physically.

But the public does have a right to hear about one of nature's greatest gifts. A wonder drug that no company or government can control or regulate, one that is always at hand and completely free!

Open your mind now and get ready to hear all about these incredible medical facts on human urine and its therapeutic value – they will change the way you live your life.

The Constituents of Urine: The Body's Own Perfect Food & Medicine

In the year1975, one of the world's leading biologists, the co-founder of Miles Laboratories, Dr. A.H. Free, published his findings on Urine Therapy in Clinical Laboratory Practice. Surprisingly, he told the truth, which would take your breath away. He revealed that urine is actually a sterile body compound that is far purer than distilled water. He also recognized that urine truly contains thousands of compounds, most of which could only be isolated by more modern tools with newer developments in biotechnology. Among the important constituents of urine mentioned in Dr. Free's incredible treatise is a list of rich nutrients that are simply astonishing. And yet, he points out that this is only the tip of the iceberg. Below is a list of these nutritional elements and the quantity of each in the total amount of urine you pass out daily.

Ascorbic acid …. 30 mg/day

Alanine, total …. 38 mg/day

Allantoin …. 12 mg/day

Arginine, total …. 32 mg/day

Amino acids, total …... 2.1 g/day

Biotin …. 35 mg/day

Bicarbonate …. 140 mg/day

Calcium …. 23 mg/day

Cystine …. 120 mg/day

Creatinine …. 1.4 mg/day

Epinephrine …. 0.01 mg/day

Dopamine …. 0.40 mg/day

Folic acid …. 4 mg/day

Glucose …. 100 mg/day

Glycine …. 455 mg/day

Glutamic acid …. 308 mg/day

Iron …. 0.5 mg/day

Inositol …. 14 mg/day

Iodine …. 0.25 mg/day

Lysine, total …. 56 mg/day

Magnesium …. 100 mg/day

Methionine, total …. 10 mg/day

Manganese …. 0.5 mg/day

Nitrogen, total …. 15 g/day

Ornithine …. 10 mg/day

Pantothenic acid …. 3 mg/day

Phosphorus, organic …. 9 mg/day

Phenylalanine …. 21 mg/day

Proteins, total …. 5 mg/day

Potassium …. 2.5 mg/day

Riboflavin …. 0.9 mg/day

Tyrosine, total …. 50 mg/day

Tryptophan, total …. 28 mg/day

Urea …. 24.5 mg/day

Vitamin B12 …. 0.03 mg/day

Vitamin B6 …. 100 mg/day

Zinc …. 1.4 mg/day

Reading over this unusual list of nutritional elements might give you some understanding as to why the reports of people surviving for long periods just by drinking only their own urine are true. I hope you did not forget that there are thousands of other elements in urine that weren't even mentioned in the list above? In reality, no food or medicine, natural or manmade, comes close to being as complete as urine, not even honey!

Now that you are beginning to understand exactly what we are dealing with, let's take a dive into some research to see what urine can really do.

Medical Proof of Urine's Incredible Power

For virtually the entire period of the 20th century, unknown to the general public, medical researchers and doctors were proving in both clinical and laboratory studies (testing) that human urine is a huge source of vital nutrients, enzymes, hormones, vitamins, and critical antibodies that cannot be replicated or derived (obtained) from any other source. They used human urine for healing heart disease, cancer, diabetes, allergies, auto-immune diseases, infertility, asthma, infections, open wounds and much, much more — yet they turned around and taught the public that human urine is a toxic waste product. This inconsistency between the public information and the medical truth regarding urine is clearly ridiculous, but unfortunately, has led to millions of deaths. How? Just do some research on the number of people dying from cancer and diabetes each year and you will understand the tragedy of it all. Still, the damage goes deeper -- people are dying horrible deaths out of ignorance!

Once, in 2015, I met a man suffering from a strange crippling incurable disease in a rural part of Africa. He had been so for 17 years and had lost all hope of ever finding a cure. I had no idea what the illness was, nor did I have access to a lab to run diagnostics so went the crude way When I advised him to drink his own urine in a therapeutic mode, he thought I was crazy. He later changed his mind and did. He was on his way to a full recovery in a week and, for the first time in 14 years, took his first steps in a short walk the second week.

But am I the first doctor to nudge patients in the right direction? Am even the first to publish or talk about it publicly? The answer both times is no. There are quite a few doctors and researchers that have walked this path, but each time, their voice and findings have been cleverly suppressed. I will mention just the ones you can look up in any medical book or journals with information dating back 70 years.

1) In 1947, just two years after World War 2, oncologist, Dr. J. Plesch, made the following publication in the Medical Press – "urine acts as an outstanding and safe, natural vaccine that has been shown to cure a wide range of disorders including hepatitis, asthma, whooping-cough, hay fever, migraines, hives, intestinal dysfunctions, and more. It is totally safe and results in no side effects."

2) Another oncologist, Dr. M. Soeda of the University of Tokyo followed this up with

another publication in 1968. He reported as follows… "a patient with intractable ovarian cancer was effectively treated with Human Urine Derivative. She is now totally cured and enjoying the rest of her life."

3) In 1983, immunologist Dr. C.W. Wilson of Law Hospital, Scotland, after conducting extensive laboratory and clinical research, stated the following: "It was quickly appreciated that undiluted human urine administered orally was quite therapeutically effective for Immune Therapy. This process was introduced when it became obvious that an allergic condition in the patient had become uncontrollable."

4) In 1962 researchers from the Harvard Medical School (Remington, Lerner & Finland) discovered that active "antibodies to typhoid, cholera, diphtheria, polio, pneumonia, salmonella and Leptospira existed in the unconcentrated urine of infected persons."

5) In 1951, a Scandinavian researcher showed that human urine has the ability to wipe out tuberculosis from the human system? This is a deadly disease that is now resistant to all antibiotics.

6) In the year1938, Dr. L. Muldavis of the Royal Free Hospital, London conducted a series of researches into open wounds and severe burns using urea (the main solid component of human urine). One of those studies, reports: "In the United States, urea has been very effectively used for the treatment of numerous infected wounds and it has proven so effective that even the deepest of wounds can be treated very effectively…. Urea treatment has actually been successful where other advanced medical treatments failed. For treatment of external staph infections, urea was found preferable to all other dressing…there are no side effects to its use.".

7) In 1954, the July issue of the Journal of the American Medical Association reported that

"More scientific papers have been published on human urine than on any other organic compound."

8) "Experience has revealed that intramuscular injections of human urine are the best methods for handling countless numbers of immunological illnesses including psoriasis, asthma, *basal cell carcinoma* and a host of other disorders." Reuter Report August 14, 1990

All these extraordinary findings were published in different medical journals, but no one ever heard about them because normal people don't go reading medical journals, only members of the medical community do. According to the American Medical Association, thousands of scientific and technical papers relating to the amazing properties of urine have been published over the last half-century. All this concern over a substance that we are all told is pure waste? Unfortunately, most of these papers have been suppressed or allowed to fade away by the medical community who read them due to the reasons outlined in the previous chapter.

Yes, all the top medical doctors and scientists know all about the amazing properties of human urine and human urine therapy but will never tell the public officially about it.

The Most Astonishing Secret About Urine That Are Hidden by The Medical Community

Below are the most fascinating secrets about human urine that are hidden from the public.

1. The Home of The Unborn Child Is Built of Urine

The most medically suppressed secret about Urine, a precious bit of information you will almost never find elsewhere, is that human infants, while developing in the womb, actually live in and breathe in urine!

The amniotic fluid that surrounds infants in the womb is majorly urine. The infant 'lives in' and "breathes in" this urine-filled amniotic fluid continually. Without this fluid, the infant's lungs don't develop.

Some doctors believe that the unique softness of the baby's skin and the strange ability of in-utero infants (babies still in the womb) to heal completely and quickly without scarring after pre-birth surgery is solely due to the amazing therapeutic properties of the urine-filled amniotic fluid.

2. A Very Special Source of Food and Medicine

When carefully checked and listed, the constituents of human urine only contain items found in the human diet. Percentages certainly differ, resulting in a substance that looks and smells differently from food, but they contain the same things; the same nutrients, vitamins and minerals. The strange thing here is that, due to its nature, the urinary constituents are so valuable to human metabolism… Details of this finding were first published in an article in the New York State Journal of Medicine in June 1980 by Dr. John R. Herman. Of course, no one ever heard of it. Why? The information was suppressed in the usual way; the leaders of the medical community who read the article allowed it fade away. It was never brought up in any seminar, conference or taught in any institution of learning.

What the learned Doctor is trying to say above, in layman's language, is that the food we eat has a unique structure that makes them rather difficult for the body to completely utilize. Hence, most of the nutrients in the food you eat are passed on straight into your bloodstream where the kidneys get ahold of them through intricate filtering processes and transforms them into something different entirely… human urine!

Food and human urine, are two physically different substances with the same constituents. However, those constituents (or chemical components) are present in different amounts, which is why the two substances look very different physically but are really the same chemically. Ironically, clinical tests and research show that the human body reacts better with urine when consumed either as food or medicine!

Interestingly, Dr. John R. Herman points out further that urine therapy flourishes in many parts of the world, even till today, but most of us have no idea about it. And yet, a large volume of knowledge is available to western scientists that clearly shows the innumerable advantages of this same urine therapy.

3. Some of The Best Drugs in The World Are Made from Human Urine

The pharmaceutical companies and their researchers will never admit it openly until you dig up the facts. They don't want you to know because it's bad for a business that currently fetches them tens of billions of dollars each year. In reality, some of those pricey wonder drugs, fertility pills and glamorized cosmetic creams are made from derivatives of human urine. In the United States where most of these drugs come from, the trick was to get the FDA to approve Urea as a valid medicinal agent that could be used in all kinds of ways, not human urine itself. In case you knew it not, urea is a major constituent of urine (take another look at the list of the constituents of urine as outlined earlier).

The External Healing Effects of Urine

Reports on the strange external benefits of human urine abound too. Medical studies, both published and otherwise, tell of remarkable cases of incurable or "stubborn", severe, chronic eczema that miraculously vanishes with the introduction of urine therapy. Because urine is both anti-bacterial and anti-viral in nature, it's ideal for treating wounds, cuts, and abrasions (scrapes) of all kinds. Rashes, athlete's foot, acne and fungal skin problems of all kinds respond dramatically and so quickly to urine compresses and soaks as well.

For use at home or emergency treatment care for all manner of wounds, poisoning, poisonous stings or bites, and even broken bones, human urine is an unrivaled, proven natural healing agent that ultimately provides prompt therapeutic benefits under any circumstances.

Straightening Out the Misconceptions

When asked what uric acid is, the average person would invariably reply that it is a toxic body waste. No, this is so wrong. The opposite is exactly the case. Human Urine, administered therapeutically, accomplishes the impossible.

In 1982, medical scientists/researchers at the prestigious University of California, Berkeley, reported the amazing discovery that "uric acid had the ability to completely destroy all cancer-causing, body-damaging free radicals and is actually one of the most important biological factors that enable (allow) human beings to live a whole lot longer than other mammals."

Now, how about urea itself? Urea is present in human urine, lots of it too. Isn't that the same toxic stuff that causes uremic poisoning? The answer is that you've been hoodwinked into abandoning the cheapest and most powerful universal cure in the history of mankind, one that will put your doctor out of business, and so quickly too!

Medical researchers discovered all of many decades ago that urea, is by no means a toxic body waste but an extremely versatile, extensive and highly effective medicinal agent (even traditional oriental doctors have known this for hundreds of years). It has already been proven in numerous medical studies and research that urea is the most powerful non-toxic viricidal agents (anti-virus) ever discovered by mankind. In one particular study, the polio and rabies virus [sic] were wiped out so efficiently and quickly by concentrated urea, that even the laconic medical researchers themselves were stunned: "Urea is a relatively inactive substance and definitely not a protoplasmic poison like most viricidal agents, it is indeed very surprising that poliomyelitis and rabies are killed so easily by concentrated urea solutions" (McKay & Schroeder, Society of Experimental Biology, 1936).

In reality, and as mentioned earlier, the substance Urea is an FDA-approved medicinal agent that researchers and

doctors utilize in an amazing variety of therapeutic modalities. Because of its extraordinary and complete anti-neoplastic (anti-tumor) properties, urea is presently being studied extensively for use in cancer treatments but is already being used in anti-cancer drugs. The urea compound drug known as Gliclazide is presently being used by some medical establishments, to great sasses, in the treatment of diabetics, both the insulin-dependent and non-insulin-dependent versions of the disease. As a powerful natural diuretic (substance that cause increased urine output by the body), urea is unmatched, and is a proven and recognized treatment in chronic cases of edema (buildup of excess fluid between body tissues) or swelling like excess cerebral (in the brain) and spinal pressure, epilepsy, meningitis, premenstrual edema and even glaucoma and a host of other delicate disorders in which excess fluid is a major problem. One astonished neurosurgeon, Dr. M. Javid of the University of Wisconsin, USA, reported the case of a patient who nearly lost her life from complications following a complex brain surgery: In his own words...
"Urea was administered to the patient intravenously as an emergency measure (injected into the bloodstream through a vein). Within 20 minutes from the beginning of injection, her blood pressure had returned to normal... From that point

on, her recovery was completely uneventful. In this particular case, urea definitely proved to be life-saving, because before its administration, the patient's survival was improbable. In many similar cases, urea was discovered to be life-saving".

The Biological Answer to A Therapeutic Mystery

The medical findings on human urine and human urine constituents are completely overwhelming, and yet most people find it so difficult to understand why the human body excretes elements that are so clearly valuable to human health and well-being. The question is best answered by taking a good look at the way in which the human kidneys function.

As blood moves through the human body's circulatory system, it ends up flowing through the kidneys at an average rate of around 1200 ml of blood per minute. Inside the kidneys (both), the blood is continuously filtered through a vast system of very minute tubules called **nephron** which sifts out (filters), not just excess water, but minerals, vitamins, enzymes, hormones, salts, and several hundreds of other elements which include vital antibodies, uric acid and urea. While a significant portion of these vital physiological elements get reabsorbed into the bloodstream, a certain amount of extremely important blood constituents is pooled up by the kidneys into a special liquid doctors technically refer to as a "plasma ultrafiltrate" (urine to the layman). A good amount of this nutrient-rich urine is still reabsorbed into the body, but some remain in the kidney for a short period of time and then get released into a tube known as the urethra, which channels the urine into the bladder from where it is finally excreted out of the body.

Now, the obvious question here is, why does the body even excrete valuable nutrients, enzymes, hormones, water, etc., that are so critical to body functions. The answer, in simple terms, is that the human kidneys are naturally programmed to excrete a specific portion of urine as a way of getting rid of certain vital elements in the blood that are simply not needed at a particular point in time. For example, you've just been out for some exercise, a mooring run, in the park. You come home all hot and sweaty, but very thirsty, and so you have two big glasses of water, drinking them straight down. Now at that point, you've probably taken in a lot more water than your body really needs. But no worries – your kidneys will fix things just perfectly by balancing up the amount of water that is delivered into your bloodstream by your abundant water drinking, and through your urine, will expel the excess amount of water completely from your body.

Now water is definitely a life-sustaining element the human body cannot do without. So why is it then excreted from our body? The answer is all too obvious. The body needs a specific amount of water to function correctly, but there are times when there's just too much of it in your system and it is then that the excess needs to be removed, and that is the job of the kidneys – regulation and control of the levels of all elements in the blood/body.

Too much of anything is a very bad thing. Too much water in the blood is deadly. Too much sugar in the body is fatal. Too much salt in the blood is simply deadly. Even vitamin C, a wonderful nutrient to the body, too high a concentration of this vitamin or any other nutrient could kill you. This is the main reason why the kidneys get rid of valuable elements from the body through urine — too much of any good thing at all isn't good for your body or health. The is exactly the case with urea.

You see, just like any other nutrient or element in the bloodstream, urea only becomes deadly when the kidneys become diseased or damaged and cannot perform their jobs correctly. Urea is one of the main constituents of human urine and so when the kidneys are damaged, faulty or diseased, the first problem the victim develops is uremic poisoning – a critical accumulation of urea in the body. And this is the reason why so many people have witnessed or heard of uremic poisoning and how deadly urea can be to the body. These people are stunned and so confused when they hear about the wonders of urine therapy or read that medical research and clinical studies show urea to be a widely-used, FDA-approved medicine. Unfortunately, there is no medically qualified person at hand to set them straight and most do no medical research whatever.

Your kidneys do not do any damage to your body by removing excess elements (nutrients), they're merely excreting the exact amount not currently needed by your body at a specific point in time. This natural rule goes for almost every nutrient, antibody, hormone, enzyme, etc., that are vital to your survival — in theory, the kidneys keep that precise amount your body needs at a particular time and excretes the amount not needed into your urine. And as doctors and medical scientists have come to discover, these urinary elements (or constituents) extracted from the body/blood can be therapeutic wonder-working bullets.

Human Urine: A Billion Dollar Industry

Regardless of what the public has been hoodwinked into believing about human urine being a poisonous body waste product, pharmaceutical companies in the USA, Canada and the UK alone earn billions of dollars each year from the sale of expensive drugs made from the constituents of human urine.

At the dawn of the new millennium, Pergonal, a fertility drug that is made from human urine, had already crossed the $1billion yearly sales mark and that figure has been on the increase on a yearly basis. Urokinase, a minor ingredient in human urine, is processed into drug form and marketed as a miracle drug, to be precise, a "miracle blood clot dissolver" for unblocking coronary arteries.

Urea, a substance that has been medically proven to be among the best moisturizers in the world, is a hit with the cosmetic industry. These multimillion dollar cosmetic companies process human urine and package it in glamorized and expensive lotions and creams.

Have you ever heard of or used Murine ear drops? Produced from carbamide, that drug is nothing but synthetic urea.

Looking at the actual facts, the tragedy of the universal disinformation campaign on human urine is exceeded only by the irony of our unknowing, and often incredibly expensive purchases of what we all wrongly, but firmly believe to be our bodies' "useless" and "offensive" waste-product... human urine!

Modern Acceptance of a Misunderstood Therapy

Due to the pervasive public misunderstanding about what human urine really is and how it can be of enormous medical benefit to us, the frequently amazing circumstantial stories of survival and healing through urine consumption and use have been regularly ignored, mocked or written off completely as "old wives' tales." However, when people get to learn about the real facts, as outlined above, these stories take on new significance that not even medical doctors are willing to ignore.

Below are some of the most tragic incidents that have opened the eyes of many over the years.

Ever watched an old movie titled "Alive"? It's the true-life story of a South American football team whose aircraft crashed in a remote region of the snow-capped Andes Mountains in the dead of winter. More than half of the football team died at the moment of the crash and the survivors, including the injured, were stranded on the spot for several months. They only survived by eating the raw flesh of their already dead friends and the ones who died later from injuries. A good part of the movie focused on two individuals whose initial wounds weren't so bad, but advanced into serious infections. Knowing no way to handle the wounds of the two, the survivors could only sympathize with them until they died. Now, what if these people had knowledge of the incredible healing powers of human urine?

On October 16, 1992, rescue workers in Egypt found a 37-year-old man alive, buried in an enclosure deep under earthquake rubble. He survived for nearly 82 hours (4 days) by merely drinking his own urine. His wife, mother and daughter, who were all with him in the enclosure, refused to do this same thing and so they died horribly. In swift reaction, the Associated Press pointed out that these women and the child would never have died had they been aware of the simple truth that not only would their own urine bring them no harm but would have provided a power-packed combination of liquid food and medicine (nutrients, vitamins and critical immune factors) that would have kept them alive, and in good health too, until help arrived.

"Four Sri Lankan Special Forces commandos who free drifted more than 1,000 miles across the Indian Ocean to Thailand in a tiny boat, after they had been in a deadly ambush and given up for dead, were given a blissful welcome when they finally returned home. According to the Military's press release, these brave men managed to survive on the tiny boat drifting aimlessly on the vast seas for weeks by catching turtles and drinking their own urine,' …. Kyodo News Service, Tokyo, Japan, July 30, 1990 "

Several years later, another story hit the news. This time, in the Philippines. A male cook was discovered alive deep in the rubble of the Hyatt Hotel, 14 days after a powerful earthquake destroyed the northern Philippines. Dry and perfectly healthy, with only minor wounds on his body, this cook told news reporters that he survived by drinking his own urine.

At a time when medical expenses and the soaring cost of drugs are widespread, a time when new bacteria and viruses are outsmarting even the best efforts of cutting-edge medicine, and natural disasters are on the increase, putting basic necessities out of the reach of all, the facts about urine therapy may well become the greatest survival lesson any person will ever learn.

24. THE SECRETS AND REALITIES OF URINE THERAPY

Urinotherapy, or urine therapy, is by far the most effective natural remedy for illnesses and diseases. It is also the safest method of treatment because it has no side effects whatever. Urine has the power to prevent, control and, yes, cure all manner of chronic diseases including Arthritis, Cancer, Diabetes, Mental Retardation, High Blood Pressure, HIV/AIDS, Kidney failure, Muscular Dystrophy, Psoriasis, and Cerebral Palsy, etc.

Urine is a very powerful Immune System booster, it improves Nervous Disorders, dissolves and then removes Toxins which have accumulated in the body over time. Urine has the unique ability to revive dead cells and tissues and this helps it rebuild the resistance power of important organs like the Heart, Brain, Lungs, Liver, Pancreas, and Intestine. This means that urine, in addition to rejuvenating our body, protects our general health, fights the aging process and increase our lifespan.

We can get rid of every last one of those chronic diseases with the natural healing powers of urine! Urine therapy is the solution for every ailment affecting our body;

there is nothing it can't cure or control, even those ailments modern medicine label as incurable are no obstacle. Urine therapy will boost, not only your health, but your self-confidence, energy levels, and fitness. The general result, always, is a happy, and disease free, long life.

If urine, or excreta as it's medically called, is half as poisonous as most medical experts claim, then why has no one died from drinking it yet? Urine Therapy will wipe out any disease or illness provided it is applied systematically and in the proper method.

Urine is the "Medicine of life", a natural liquid that can cure a host of diseases. A gift of nature for the sole purpose of sustaining health and life, which leads to longevity and happiness. Urine has no equal in the world and, like sunlight, air and water, cannot be reproduced through any other alternative method, whether traditional or scientific.

For those who doubt the existence of a creator, urine should clear your mind. This **water of life** is definitely a natural gift from an all-knowing creator who foresaw the terrible suffering of mankind in face of incurable diseases and old age. Urine therapy combines spiritual growth and physical well-being to bring about perfect health. Urine, "the healing power within you", is the only real way you can save yourself from incurable chronic disease, illnesses, and overall bad health. Nothing else and no one else can help you – unless, of course, you can help and heal yourself.

Urine, as a Universal Remedy for all distempers (viral animal diseases that affect different kinds of animals i.e. rabies) inside and outside the human body, is simply awesome. Urine acts as an antidote for poisons; destroys all poisons and every disease resulting from VIT, KAFFA, PITT. But that's not all! Urine actually improves digestion, the body's energy levels and overall strength. Urine cures all these chronic diseases and enhances body functions by flushing out piled up waste products and toxins from the body and stimulating its defensive mechanism in a unique way. Faced with the poisonous bites of insect and other such animals, urine works more wonders.

Are you a pregnant woman suffering for one manner of complication or another? Are you a woman who just has excessive menstruation or a tumor in the Uterus? Urine will amaze you with what it can do! Urine does battle with everything, from diseases of the eyes to cancerous cells and worms that live in the intestines, scarlet fever, typhoid fever and all skin diseases.

Urine therapy can simply be defined as good health and long life in glassfuls; an entirely drugless and painless healing system. It purifies the blood, improves health and adds years to your life. Urine, in addition to unique antibiotics and protein, contains all the essential compounds, Hormones, Vitamins, minerals, salts and chemical compounds, which are crucial for optimal growth and body maintenance. The volatile salts of Urine neutralize powerful acids and radicals present in our system, thereby destroying the foundations of most diseases in the human body.

The number one obstacle in the way of newbies to urine therapy is the taste and color of urine. Consider this: when you wash very dirty laundry, the residual water is disgusting but in the case of clean laundry with mere stains, the residual water is neat. The point? The color and taste of your urine depends entirely upon what you eat and drink and the kind of illnesses brewing inside your body. When you have things like bad oils, salt and all kinds of rubbish in your diet, the color of your urine will be yellow and the smell will be terrible. If you have bacterial or fungal based diseases brewing inside of you, the taste of your urine will be so bitter, you'll probably puke and be put off urine therapy for life. Endeavor to overcome this stigma of the terrible taste and smell of your own urine, for you are the cause of it. For people with a habit of eating poor diets who urgently need to switch to urine therapy, I have devised a solution called the '**trigger method**' – we will deal with this subject in full later.

Avoid poor foods at all costs. If you are going into urine therapy, learn to eat balanced and light diets, drink lots of water and nutrient rich juices, this is the only way you will pass colorless and tasteless urine, which will look and taste much like ordinary water but is packed with minerals, vitamins, and, depending on what illness is affecting you, unique antibiotics and proteins to kick start the therapy.

The Universal Cure

As mentioned earlier, there are an estimated 8,000 diseases in the world today and that number keeps increasing daily, with new strains appearing in different regions. Medicine, orthodox and unorthodox, offer so many different methods of treatment for just a fraction of these ailments. Most of these treatments have limited effects on the diseases while others have too many side effects. Bottom line, modern and traditional medicine are overwhelmed by the multitude and complexity of mankind's health predicaments. Below are some of these diseases that have defied cure and the way urine therapy deals with them.

Diabetes

The number of people suffering from diabetes worldwide crossed the half a billion mark at the end of 2016. In the United States alone, at least 1 out of every 9 people has one form of diabetes or the other (over 30 million people), with the disease ranking as the 6th highest killer in that country. In China and India, the case is a lot worse!

Diabetes is the root cause of numerous chronic diseases and it has defied cure. The only proven way to treat, control and eventually cure diabetes is Urine Therapy. It is the easiest and safest method and it cuts out all the other resulting complicating illness such as heart disease, hypertension, kidney failure and diabetic retinopathy.

HIV/AIDS

This highly infectious disease, which slowly destroys the immune system, does not respond to any medication.

HIV infections result in the progressive reduction of the number of T cells of CD 4 counts in the immune system. Due to this deficiency, the person's immunity to illnesses and diseases gradually begins to decrease. The person's overall health deteriorates on a daily basis and various other illnesses set in. The response of doctors here is to treat the compounding illnesses with other medicine and then try to slow down the deterioration of the immune system with Anti-Retroviral Therapy (ART). Nonetheless, the patient's sufferings worsen as there is no known cure for HIV/AIDS... mind you, this is according to modern medicine.

The ultimate healing magic of Urine Therapy is far more powerful than the mere delaying effect of Anti-Retroviral Therapy. Urine therapy brings the entire health deterioration problem in HIV/AIDS patients under firm control and improves the body's energy levels. With this control in full force and other complications held at bay, urine then proceeds to fight the very virus that caused the whole problem in the first place, the Human Immune Deficiency Virus – and this leads to the eventual cure of HIV/AIDS in people. Urine therapy strengthens the immune system and gradually begins to stimulate the increase of the CD 4 Counts. In some reported cases, people with CD 4 counts as low as 50 have seen it increase to 800 and above within a very short time. Just imagine the physical improvement this implies!

Cerebral Palsy

This brain disorder (deficiency of Motor Control) is caused by brain damage around the time of birth and marked by involuntary spasms and lack of muscle control, particularly in the limbs People who suffer from this disease are afflicted with twisted legs and hands which they cannot move or balance without assistance (paralysis). In addition, they often cannot hear, speak, sit or stand.

Urine has the power to cure or control all ailments resulting from birth related issues and Cerebral Palsy is no exception. Children afflicted with this disease will be cured if subjected to special urine therapy that calls for the use of their own urine only after a certain period of time (this point is explained later). Since urine, in addition to reviving cells, enhances all manner of brain functions including memory and intelligence, these children will have their physical deformity fixed to a major extent, if not completely. Their twisted limbs (hands and legs) will become straight and strong in time, muscle mass will develop in the right place and their body will look normal.

Arthritis

Urine does battle with all manner of arthritis. It doesn't matter how many years you've had it or how bad it has become, when hit with urine, particularly your own urine, in therapeutic mode, it must go. With rheumatoid arthritis that can afflict young people, once you start drinking your own urine, the illness should start disappearing within 3 days. Yes, you heard right. 3 days!

Why Is Urine Therapy So Powerful Against Dieses?

Urine is packed with all the vital chemical compounds required for the optimal growth and maintenance of the human body. This unique quality is unrivaled by any other medicine or procedure and this makes urine the best natural tonic ever known to man. Urine contains some volatile salts, which are highly beneficial because they engage harmful acids and free radicals in the body, thus destroying the building blocks of most diseases and sicknesses before they take hold.

Diseases and sickness, whether internal or external, are no match for urine. Urine destroys everything from poisons to viruses living in the blood. Urine strengthens the immunes system and revitalizes the cells. It gives new life, brings new energy, sanitizes blood and deep cleans the skin, getting rid of all manner of problems. Urine lays waste to disease and defects of the eyes, improves the process of digestion and destroys all lung infections from simple colds to cough. Urine has the unique ability to repair and reconstruct all the vital organs of the body from basic levels including the brain, lungs, liver, heart, pancreas, and kidneys. Urine is also very effective in the dental, and oral department.

The drinking of urine is a guaranteed cure for the following diseases – kidney diseases, liver diseases, bile troubles, dropsy, sinuses stoppages, lung diseases, jaundice, plague and other such poisonous fevers, all manner of STDs and blood sugar problems which lead to diabetes. When applied outwardly, urine deep cleans the skin, destroys all manner of complex skin diseases, removes all kinds of rashes, cures dandruff, excellently fights a host of other diseases from wrinkles to athlete's foot.

Urine is actually the watery aspect of the blood in a unique form, and so one person's urine can literally be drunk by another with excellent results. This process is very important in situations where a sick person cannot produce enough urine of his or her own – or cannot produce any at all – to drink and so cure his or her body of the afflicting disease. The urine of a healthy person can be drunk (or massaged into the skin) by any other person who has difficulty in producing enough of his or her own Urine. This unique process is similar to the donation of blood but much simpler. Provided a person is healthy and eats the right foods, he or she can donate urine to just about anyone.

A mother can donate her urine to her child for drinking, a man to a friend or stranger. The only rules are that the urine must be extremely fresh, it must be drunk immediately after being passed by the donor, and most importantly, it must be clean, colorless, and odorless – all of which indicates a healthy donor on balanced diets.

This particular method of urine donation is so helpful with children and other people afflicted with diseases such as **Cerebral Palsy** and other mental disorders that make it unsafe to drink their own urine from the beginning of the therapy. This method is also important for people who are unable to drink their own urine while undergoing treatment for some kinds of chronic diseases, especially those who have been diagnosed with Terminal cancer – urine can help them but not their own urine, which is probably radioactive as a result of radioactive treatments received. People undergoing treatments for afflictions related to certain poison cannot drink their own urine too, became the first thing the body will be doing at the introduction of the overwhelming urine therapy, will be flushing out all that poison as quickly as it can through the urine.

So, you see, until you study and understand the laws of urine therapy, do not embark on it, particularly if you are turning to it to cure a chronic disease. There are set patterns you must follow to achieve the desired results; patterns laid down by the chronicles of traditional experts who have treated so many people with ailments similar to yours. Since modern medicine refuses to recognize urine therapy, unique knowledge of it is carried on from generation to generation. Today, a lot of that knowledge can be found freely in special books like this one.

Read on….

Clear Benefits of Urine Therapy

1. Urine therapy is the most effective and most powerful natural remedy for illnesses and diseases and it has no equal, natural or artificial.

2. Urine possesses unique healing powers which enable it Control and Cure all types of Chronic Diseases.

3. Urine has the power to improve Nervous Disorders, boost the Immune System, dissolve and flush out accumulated Toxins in the body.

4. Urine has the ability to revive dead cells and tissues, thereby rebuilding the diseases resistant powers of important organs such as the Heart, Brain, Pancreas, Lungs, Intestine, and Liver.

5. Urine revitalizes the body and protects its overall Health.

6. Urine is one of the safest methods of treatment known to man and it does not have any side effects.

7. Urine therapy is an entirely drugless and efficient method of healing all types of Chronic Diseases.

8. With regards to cancer treatment, urine is more powerful and beneficial than Radiation and Chemotherapy.

9. Urine has the ability to destroy cancerous cells without harming other healthy cells.

10. Urine can drastically reduce the unwelcome side effects of Chemotherapy treatments in cancer patients.

11. For terminal patients afflicted with Chronic Disease, urine is another chance at life.

12. Without any doubt, urine therapy is the best method of treatment for diseases and it has awesome results compared to all other alternative therapies.

25. URINE THERAPY: INCURABLE DISEASES, AND STDs

This chapter outlines how urine therapy can control or induce healing for some horrible diseases that have defied modern medicine.

Best Practices

Considering urine therapy as an alternative to your illness or disease? The following are the best practices for you.

1. People in certain regions of the Orient instantly turn to urine therapy once they are diagnosed with the incurable disease, cancer.

Urine Therapy is very efficient in the control and eventual cure of cancer. It is much more effective and beneficial than either Radiation or Chemotherapy. Urine therapy has the ability to wipe out Cancerous Cells effectively, preventing the spread of the disease to other parts of the body. It kills all the poisonous material in the cancerous cell without creating any side effect and so ensures the safety of other healthy cells.

For those requiring blood transfusion, urine therapy is a very safe and effective remedy.

2. People afflicted with all manner of Chronic Disease should turn to Urine Therapy early enough for treatment.

Drinking Urine, massaging it into the affected areas of the body or placing wet urine packs on, can help; it's usually part of the therapy. To help in the manufacture of more and cleaner urine, drink lots of water and nutrient rich juices, eat light diets that are well-balanced nutritionally – see the list of best foods discussed in earlier chapters of this book to take your pick.

3. Get Completely Adapted to Urine Therapy

Adaption to Urine Therapy allows one undergo what is called 'Strict Urine Fasting' which can last for 3 to 7 days. Basically, this is drinking only Urine and water throughout a particular period of treatment. The process can be repeated after a period of time to achieve even better and faster overall results.

Urine Therapy and Cancer

It is a very well-known and accepted fact that the three conventional cancer treatment methods – Surgery, Radiation therapy and Chemotherapy – are full of unwelcome side effects.

The most accepted treatment method of the three, Chemotherapy, has the potential to kill off cancerous cells in an affected area and contain its spread by killing other such cells in other parts of the body. It can also reduce the size of tumors in the body markedly.

Unfortunately, chemotherapy has quite a few unwelcome side effects. It is not selective, and so kills and destroys other healthy cells along with the Cancerous cells. Numerous complications arise as a result of this side effects and one of them is hair loss, another is chronic stomach aches and yet another is vomiting – infections, terrible muscle, and nerves pains, decrease of red and white blood cells – all of this are very unwelcome side effects indeed.

Urine Therapy, on the other hand, doesn't have any side effects – absolutely zero! It will wipe the cancer from your system and make you healthier.

Interestingly, post-surgery patients preparing to undergo Chemotherapy may inject Urine Therapy into the treatment for better results in shorter periods. It is quite possible for patients to undergo Chemotherapy as medically advised and still continue with Urine Therapy at the same time. This helps reduce the side effects of Chemotherapy with the added benefit of fast recovery. It will also boost the immune system of the patient, replenishing destroyed red and white blood cells with new and healthier once that have increased resistance abilities to the cancer itself. Basically, Urine Therapy will increase the lifespan of those cancer patients, even as it delivers them from all manner of sufferings.

Warning! Anyone undergoing Chemotherapy must not drink his or her own urine.

Patients undergoing Chemotherapy must drink the Urine of any other healthy person if they opt to follow up on Urine therapy during the treatment. Despite coming from another person, the urine will still work perfectly to reduce the numerous complications arising from the side effects of Chemotherapy. Only 36 to 48 hours after undergoing Chemotherapy, is it safe for patients to drink their own urine, provided they keep consuming lots of water. These patients may begin to drink their own urine once they find it is clear, colorless and odorless.

Neither Oncologists nor other doctors will recommend Chemotherapy or any other anti-cancer treatment to patients diagnosed with advanced and terminal stage-4 cancer. The theory is that the patient's chances of survival are way too low to withstand the terrible side effects of Chemotherapy. Doctors effectively kill the last hopes of these patients and prescribe them palliative medication (special pain relievers) to manage the pain till they eventually die.

In certain cases, there exists the opinion of palliative Chemotherapy, but just like palliative medicine, this merely reduces the pain and overall discomfort to tolerable levels. Although this helps the patients live easier, it solves nothing.

People sentenced to death in this manner (sorry to be that blunt), should switch swiftly to Urine Therapy. Remember that urine is a miracle tonic and so a condition of advanced and terminal Cancer where normal medicine does not work, is no obstacle at all. When fresh Urine hits that 'advanced and terminal stage-4 cancer body' in full therapeutic mode, the immune system will start responding in no time. Urine will prevent the cancerous cells from spreading further to other parts of the body and then kill them all off selectively, replacing all cells and tissues with better and strong ones. In very little time, the patient will be free of sufferings and their health will begin to improve markedly.

Palliative Chemotherapy is by no means powerful enough to do much good for terminal stage cancer patients. It does not cure cancer and its other benefits are limited as opposed to its numerous side effects. This mild injection shrinks Cancer cells, yes, but that's about it. Interestingly, when Palliative Chemotherapy is used along with Urine therapy, the result is a cure for Cancer.

Urine Therapy, in addition to diminishing the side effects of the Palliative injections given to Stage-4 cancer patients, will eventually cure the disease.

Points to Note About Urine Therapy and Western Medicine

1. Doctors will never recommend urine therapy for any chronic or terminal disease they cannot cure because most people see it as disgusting and won't even consider it at first. In addition, urine therapy is well outside the legal limits of modern (orthodox) medicine, and as such, any official recommendation of it can bring the doctor legal

problems among many other things. What doctors do instead, is manage the illness till the patient's death.

2. In many cases, patients may completely avoid chemotherapy and surgery if they adapt Urine Therapy at the early stages of the disease. As long as the right method of treatment is followed properly, the results will present itself.

Illnesses, Anti-Aging, Urine Therapy Dosage and Triggers

Below are some illnesses and diseases and how to treat them with urine therapy. These are for beginners and it will be made as simple as possible.

Triggers are required in urine therapy for two reasons. Firstly, to ensure that your body passes out the right kind of urine for you to consume (or drink). Secondly, certain diseases respond faster to urine therapy with the presence of certain foods or supplements in your system. For example, drinking your urine directly or rubbing it on your skin when you have a bacterial disease like gonorrhea will give you big problems beginning with the terrible bitter taste and smell to sore throat and skin rashes it will later result in. You need a trigger to condition your urine swiftly and get past all that initial problem. Triggers are to be consumed at least one hour before the intake of the first cup of urine, in certain cases a whole day ahead.

The most important step to take before you begin urine therapy, therefore, is to change your diet to a healthy and well-balanced one. Get rid of the alcohol, stop smoking already, get rid of the buggers, French fries, doughnuts, sugars and heavy oils. Turn to a balanced light diet right away and you won't regret it. Check out the previous chapters on foods and supplements to consume in other to achieve optimal health.

* Living A long, Disease Free and Healthy life

Prevention, they say, is better than cure. To live a disease free and healthy long life, we need to fully harass the awesome anti-aging benefits of urine. To achieve this, drink 3 glassfuls of your own urine daily for the rest of your life. With proper daily diets that are rich in nutrient-packed foods such as fruits and vegetables, it is possible to reduce dosage after a while to just two cups a day or even one, particularly if you are the office worker kind who's too busy to keep rushing to the toilet to get a drink!

Trigger: The trigger needed here are fruits and vegetable. To be safe, eat them solely as food for a whole day before embarking on urine therapy.

*Constant Headaches and pains

This should disappear quickly enough, never to be a problem again, with the above dosage. For an immediate fix, 3 cups of urine daily for 2 days will take care of things. In chronic cases, it's probably a sign of another illness, continue as long as symptoms persist.

Trigger: Eat some fruits, or a spoonful of honey, at least twenty minutes before your first cup of urine.

*Coughs and Cold

Drink 3 glassfuls of your own urine daily. This sickness, even in chronic conditions, should vanish within 2 or 3 days.

Trigger: Honey water or a spoonful of honey. Take it one hour before you begin urine therapy and each morning till symptom disappear.

*Clear and sharp eyesight

Eat well of diets rich in fresh green leafy vegetables, carrots, onions and honey water, and drink three glassfuls of the urine you pass daily. Put drops of the urine in your eyes daily, as often as possible for 7 days. Changes should come within the first 24 hours. For permanent results, use urine as a daily eye drop all your life.

Trigger; Carrots and onions. Eat well of these two vegetables before beginning the therapy.

*STDs – To treat gonorrhea, for beginners, it is wise to first eat a lime orange before you start with the therapy then take one every day after that for at least 7 days – do it on alternate days if you like. Take 3 glassfuls of your urine daily for fourteen days. Drinking all or 90% of your urine daily, you should be fine in 7 days.

Trigger: 1 Lime orange a day

*Syphilis – Everything here is the same as with gonorrhea but the dosage is 3 glassfuls a day for 1 month. Drinking all the urine you pass out, you should be fine in 14 to 21 days.

*Cancers – For this disease, it's best you turn fully to urine therapy and stay with it. Eat a diet rich in cancer-fighting food (listed above), then drink every drop of the urine you pass out until symptoms disappear completely –

this method is for faster results. Once cured, relax to 5 glassfuls of your urine a day and don't stop for at least one week. Continue with 3 glasses of urine daily for the rest of your life for good health.

If you begin fighting cancer with 3 glassfuls of urine a day, it will take longer for it to get cured.

*HIVE'/AIDS – This is one of the most difficult diseases to cure. Urine therapy here takes from 3 to 6 months. Dosage – 3 to 6 glassfuls of fresh urine for 6 or 3 months respectively. Drink every drop of your urine for faster results in 3 months. Always keep your diet light and very healthy. Pack it full of some of the foods mention earlier in this book, the supplements too. Your body will need all the boost it can get because it's going to war!

Trigger: I believe there is a special trigger for this illness that can wipe it out more effectively and faster. I'm doing some private research on the subject at the moment.

*Skin Infections and Rashes

There are too many different kinds of skin infections, viral and bacterial. One thing they all have in common is that urine does battle with them all. The way you use urine therapy for skin infections is a bit different, though. You apply it directly to the affected area with soaks and compresses. Eat lots of citrus fruits like oranges, lemon and lime so your urine will be awash with highly charged bacteria and virus fighting nutrients.

Conclusion

Three glassfuls of fresh urine daily is the average dosage in urine therapy necessary to cure most sicknesses and diseases. Keep your diet balanced and this will give you complete good health, youthfulness and longer life. Decades will literally be knocked off your life and your anti-aging war will be won!

Urine is the most powerful and most versatile anti-aging substance ever known.

For faster results with urine therapy, you have to drink more urine. That's how it works. The more urine you drink, the faster the result and this is why some people go into urine fasting wherein they drink every drop of their own urine and water. One very clever secret is to carefully add fruits and vegetable to that strict fasting diet or better still, use the miracle tonic – honey water.

Now you have all the knowledge you need to slow down the aging process in your body perfectly and increase your lifespan. Knowledge is power. Put the power to work today and live longer from tomorrow.

Thank you for reading my book. If you found the information in it useful, won't you please take a moment to leave me a review at your favorite retailer?

Thank you!

Dr. Laura Zeaman (Author)

ABOUT THE AUTHOR

Dr. Laura Zeaman is a semi-retired American doctor with over 7 years of working experience in Europe and Africa. She is an advocate of natural health and healing and has published several books on the subject.

For Laura, writing is more of a hobby now and she currently lives a quiet life with her husband and three kids in California, USA.

OTHER BOOKS FROM THIS AUTHOR

- Breastfeeding Made Simple for The First Time Moms
- Ancient and Modern Secrets of Health and Long Life
- Urine Colors and What They Say About Your Health.
- How to Bring Back Excursive into Your Life
- Brain Food and Brain Health
- Perfect Vision for Life
- The Health Benefits of Onions

To find a full listing of the author's books please visit the author's book page on the publisher's website:

Author's book page:
https://www.kingreads.com/tag/author-laura-zeaman-books/

ABOUT THE PUBLISHER

Kingreads is a book publishing and promotions team that works strictly with talented authors and individuals with good ideas to publish.

Find more books our website: **kingreads.com**

View Our author list:

https://www.kingreads.com/authors/

Kingreads: *We publish only the best books.*

NOTES

Made in United States
North Haven, CT
12 June 2022